MINDFULNESS SEX

Better sex to nurture love and to reach sexual health in the couple. How to build a relationship with awareness, mindful loving and sex. Sexual magic and magnetism power of love.

DONNA DARE

© Copyright 2019 - All rights reserved.

The content contained within this book may not be reproduced, duplicated or transmitted without direct written permission from the author or the publisher.
Under no circumstances will any blame or legal responsibility be held against the publisher, or author, for any damages, reparation, or monetary loss due to the information contained within this book. Either directly or indirectly.

Legal Notice:
This book is copyright protected. This book is only for personal use. You cannot amend, distribute, sell, use, quote or paraphrase any part, or the content within this book, without the consent of the author or publisher.

Disclaimer Notice:
Please note the information contained within this document is for educational and entertainment purposes only. All effort has been executed to present accurate, up to date, and reliable, complete information. No warranties of any kind are declared or implied. Readers acknowledge that the author is not engaging in the rendering of legal, financial, medical or professional advice. The content within this book has been derived from various sources. Please consult a licensed professional before attempting any techniques outlined in this book.
By reading this document, the reader agrees that under no circumstances is the author responsible for any losses, direct or indirect, which are incurred as a result of the use of information contained within this document, including, but not limited to, — errors, omissions, or inaccuracies.

Table of Contents

Description 1
Introduction 4
Chapter 1: The Psychology of Sex 9
    Climate of Intimacy 10
    The Female Sexual Map 13
    The Female as Identity 13
    The Clitoris 15
Chapter 2: Sex and Spirituality 18
Chapter 3: Prepare Mind and Body for Sex 24
    Peace and privacy 24
    Feather the nest 26
    It's up to you to lubricate or not 26
    Bath or shower 27
Chapter 4: Keep Your Enemy Closer 29
Chapter 5: Reconnect With Your Partner 48
Chapter 6: Breathing and Diaphragmatic Breathing 61
    Breathing 62
Chapter 7: Setting the Mood 68
    Peace and privacy 68
    Feather the nest 70
    It's up to you to lubricate or not 70
    Bath or shower 71

Chapter 8: Spin Your Chakras and Breathe To Ecstasy 73
Chapter 9: Sexual Domination and Submission 76
Chapter 10: Reel Life to Real Life 88
Chapter 11: Personal Lubricants 94
   Slippin' and a slidin' – the lubrication basics 95
   Where to buy it 99
Chapter 12: So you want to be a Superhero? 102
Chapter 13: Develop Sexual Intuition 108
Chapter 14: Sexual Massages 115
   Types of massage to try on your partner 119
Chapter 15: Mindful Oral Sex 123
Chapter 16: Alternative Sexual Experiences 135
Chapter 17: Would You Ever? 148
   Role play 149
   Bondage 152
   Spanking 153
Conclusion 155

Description

Things are not always exactly the same, and marriage is not an exception. However, change is not always a bad thing. Even in the worst scenarios where you think things are going downhill or changing for worse, there is still an opportunity to turn them around. You must remember that everything has a solution, including even the worst scenarios. Most problems that you will face through marriage can be solved, but in order for this to happen, both parties need to be willing to try and do their best. Patience is the key. Don't expect things to work out in your first attempt. If they do, that's great, but if they don't, that's not a reason to stop. You need to keep trying until it works, no matter how many times you need to try. As with many other things, we have to try our best instead of giving up easily. It is only by giving the best of us that we can reach our goal and even when you have reached your goal, keep trying your best.

Marriage is a continuous process, so we need to try to be better at it every day. It is not enough with the "I do" you said a while ago; it is not enough with living together, having children or signing papers. In order to have a strong relationship, you need to continue to create positive experiences and a healthy environment. You need to keep working on your relationship, making each other feel good, important, desired, etc. There are so many ways to make your relationship stay alive and make each other feel special: a kiss, a touch, saying something nice, writing down a poem or message, doing something special for one another; those are things that are so easy to do and can be done often. Not everything has to be very elaborate and cost money. In fact, sometimes the smallest things can be the most meaningful. So, there are no excuses; no matter what gets in the way, there is always something we can do.

This guide will focus on the following:

- The psychology of sex
- Sex and spirituality
- Prepare mind and body for sex
- Keep your enemy closer
- Reconnect with your partner
- Breathing and diaphragmatic breathing
- Spin your chakras and breathe to ecstasy
- Develop sexual intuition
- Sexual massages
- Mindful oral sex

- Alternative sexual experiences... AND MORE!!!

Always look for different ways to help you and your partner work on your relationship.

Introduction

Romance stems from intimacy, as it is ultimately an extension of the intimacy itself. When there is intimacy in a relationship, you can be certain that some level of romance will prevail. If you want to have a really exciting sex life, you will want to build a solid foundation of intimacy and frost it off with a healthy helping of romance. Regardless of what someone's intimacy preference is, they will most certainly want to experience romance in their life. You can decide how you will display romance based on their preference for types of intimacy.

For Physical People

Anyone who likes physical intimacy will want to experience acts of romance in the physical sense. There are many ways that you can be romantic towards someone physically. When you are physically romantic, you want to do so with both sexual and non-sexual intentions. What that means is that while sometimes you are going to want to allow the romance to lead towards sex, you should not always allow for it to go that far. When you use physical intimacy to result in sex every single time, it can actually break down the value of this type of intimacy as your partner will begin to predict that every time you display physical romance, you want sex. You always want to keep your partner on edge and guessing. You can do this by mixing it up and sometimes going all the way and other times holding back and letting the passion build for a few days until you allow it to evolve into sexual romance.

Even if your partner likes physical romance, it doesn't mean they will like all physical touches. They may prefer some over others. Again, communication is the key to finding out what your partner likes. However, these are great places to start:

- Sensual massages
- Caressing or stroking
- Hugging
- Holding hands
- Cuddling or holding
- Kissing the face
- Kissing the lips

For Emotional People

For anyone who likes emotional intimacy, they will prefer acts of romance that stir up emotions inside of them. While physical touch will be one aspect of this, there are much more. In fact, in most cases, one of the other methods will be more likely to stir up the romance than physical touching will. Again, you want to use your actions as an opportunity to romance your partner whether you want to have sex or not. Especially with emotional people, using acts of romance only to have sex can lead to a greater sense of hurt feelings and it can actually heavily damage the intimacy between you and your partner, thus destroying the romance. If you want to succeed, you need to be willing to be romantic without sexual intentions on a regular basis, as well as romantic with sexual intentions from time to time.

If your partner likes emotional romance, you need to be certain that your romantic actions are always genuine. Those who are turned on by their emotions are often equally turned off by their emotions, and this can quickly destroy things in your relationship. Never commit an act of romance if it isn't genuinely coming from your heart. If you are, however, acting from your heart, the following ideas are a great place to start:

- Poetry
- Telling about how you feel
- Saying "I love you."

- Showing you care through words and actions
- Romantic gestures such as flowers or chocolate
- Remembering important things about them
- Looking into their eyes to establish an emotional connection

Stirring up the romance in your relationship is important if you want to have a strong sex life. Before you start focusing on new sex positions and how to spice up sex itself, you want to build a strong foundation. A relationship that is strong with intimacy and romance is one where sex will be uninhibited and much more enjoyable for both parties. It is important that you put in the groundwork to ensure that your relationship is strong outside of sex if you want to have mind-blowing sex that is incredible every single time.

In order to strengthen our marriage, we need balance; a balance in our sexual, romantic and physical connection. All of these things are important and they are connected one way or the other. So, if one is being affected, the others can eventually struggle as well. Don't believe that as time passes, we don't need to keep trying to please our partners; our needs will always remain the same. So instead of forgetting about these 3 aspects, we need to often nourish them. For couples who have a healthy relationship, it doesn't matter how long they have been together, they still enjoy each other's company and every day still feel like an adventure. If this is what you want to achieve, you need to leave all the bad things behind and enjoy your spouse. Make every day count. Make all the good things that happen in your relationship the reason to keep going, while you make the bad ones an experience, and a story of separation. Make every day feel like the day you found out you were in love with that person.

Chapter 1: The Psychology of Sex

The vision and attitude towards life vary greatly according to the person. Similarly, they tend to be different between women and men, which are especially reflected in sexual intercourse.

For her to show a positive disposition towards sex, no matter how uninhibited it may be, she needs to feel desired and excited. If she does not feel desired and stimulated by man, her instincts will be withdrawn. Indeed, due to the disparity of cultural values between them, the woman tends to believe that if it is not required. It must be because she is not attractive enough or she is not a good lover. All this inevitably influences your erotic behavior.

When influenced by society as competitive as the current one and one which gives so much importance to the aesthetic model, her libido usually decreases. This happens because the woman wants to be perfect and if she does not respond exactly to the pattern placed by society, her self-esteem decreases. It is important to be clear that, on the one hand, men also feel insecurity in intimacy and, on the other, that the attraction she awakens does not depend exclusively on the perfection of her body. Sensuality is a sum of factors in which certain inexplicable chemistry plays a primary role.

While a man may seem very attractive to her, it is not always something physical because emotionally mature women tend to lean toward the whole personality. Ironically, men rarely understand this. Contrary to what they may suppose, the woman does not go in search of the most expert lover but of the one who, in making love, makes her feel truly desirable.

Similarly, her feminine sensibility warns her when he goes to the easy stimuli with the fixed idea of penetration without attending to her desires. This causes her to become inhibited, and ultimately, stop participating. To really enjoy sensuality, it is not possible to set aside certain specific psychological aspects since after a difficult day at home or at work, if you are tired and full of tensions, it is rare to have a good disposition for sex. The same happens if a season of stress or emotional conflict is happening.

Climate of Intimacy

To be open to frank dialogue, imagination and fantasy are the ideal elements to create a perfect climate for intimacy between lovers. When two people get carried away by the enjoyment of the senses, natural complicity is born between them which is conducive to erotic play. The woman craves to be perfect and if she does not respond exactly to the established guidelines, she feels low self-esteem. Frank dialogue and openness to imagination and fantasy are the ideal elements to create a climate conducive to intimacy.

Female sexuality has a slow awakening, needs to be stimulated for a longer time, so she is pleased to be in the arms of the sensitive man, who respects her rhythm until passion arises. If the bodies are allowed to respond freely to their desires, to embrace and stimulate themselves without the urgency of orgasm being interposed, they enjoy each and every one of the seasons of pleasure. This climate of intimacy grows surrounded by external stimuli such as a pleasant temperature, a scented atmosphere of incense, or illuminated with scented candles.

All this helps lovers to relax and positively predispose to enjoy each other. Each of the senses is important in the moment of passion: the color of the garments of the underwear or the sheets and other decorative elements excite the sensory world. Like any ceremony, sex requires a stage and rites that enrich it. It requires more and more exciting ingredients to stop it from falling into monotony. Gradually, an intimate culture is born among lovers who, as mutual knowledge grows, feel freer and more eroticized in each new encounter.

In addition to the skin that awakens with caresses, kisses, and rubs that are in themselves, messages of desire, the voice constitutes a vehicle of great sensuality because he and she enjoy creating their own unique language that increases their passion to unknown limits. Women and men do not express themselves sensually in the same way. That is why shared intimacy is the best ally for them to know and acquire confidence in their erotic games, pampering their senses, and above all, telling them what they want to give and receive to feel the maximum sexual pleasure.

Some sexologists argue that the inner frontal wall of the vagina is an erogenous zone, called the G-spot, and it is very sensitive to stimulation and is highly capable of climaxing. However, the idea is not entirely clear, and many women never discover it. Also, the idea that the hymen is preserved whole in virgin women is nothing more than one of many popular myths.

The Female Sexual Map

The genital apparatus of women is mostly hidden, except for the vulva, which is also not visible, since it is inside the thighs between the pubis or mount of Venus and the perineum. Pubic hair, in turn, hides the major and minor lips, the clitoris, the urinary orifice, and the entrance to the vagina. Its location further lowers the knowledge that women have of themselves.

To get acquainted with the genitals, it will be enough to look at them with the help of a mirror and see how the vulva is, what texture and thickness the outer and inner lips have, and what size and shape the clitoris and the cap that covers it is. It will also be helpful to discover the color, touch, and temperature of that intimate area. Some women are excited to see it, which is completely natural and pleasant but, above all, knowing each other thoroughly is the first step towards a healthy and rewarding sexuality.

The Female as Identity

In addition to being a powerful erotic claim, the hair that covers the mount of Venus and the labia of the vulva has the function of protecting the delicate anatomy of the female genitals. The skin of these fleshy lips is similar to that of the entire body. They measure about 7 or 8 centimeters in length. The labia minora are elongated - sometimes very small, sometimes so large that they appear between the exteriors - and their tissue is much more delicate and of a faint pink color. They are very sensitive to manual arousal, hence their importance in sexuality. These labia minora converge on the clitoris.

The lubricating flows that secrete the glands of the female genital area are responsible for their characteristic smell, which often results in great eroticism for men. On the other hand, many women are insecure because they fear it is unpleasant. At its entrance, the vagina is covered by a thin membrane, the hymen, which partially or completely closes it. The idea that this one is conserved whole in the virgin women is not more than one of the so many popular myths. Actually, the hymen, which is very elastic, remains in some sexually active women while in others who have never even practiced intercourse, it can be accidentally broken given its fragility.

The inside of the vagina is shaped like a canal and can be between 9 and 12 centimeters long. Its walls rub against each other, except when dilated during sexual intercourse. It is a humid, warm, and extraordinarily flexible area to allow penetration or the time of birth since during that, it reaches almost 12 centimeters in diameter. Being hidden, it tends to hormones that give the individual aspects of the color of pubic hair to the feminity of the genital tract. Through the fallopian tubes, these are formed from the lips and the clitoris, the depth, and diameter of the canal connect with the uterus, where the fertilized embryos lodge and develop. The uterus can be felt if the fingers are inserted to the bottom of the vagina. A man's penis can also touch it if it is of sufficient length or if the vaginal canal is short.

The Clitoris

A short ligament joins the pelvic bone with a fleshy bump, which is usually compared to a small penis, called a clitoris, leaving it almost hidden between the labia minora of the vulva. The portion that remains insight is the glans, which is of flexible consistency and is pink in color. Due to its vulnerability, it is protected by a membrane or cap that fulfills functions similar to those of the foreskin. Like the phallus, the clitoris has a spongy and erectile tissue inside that fills with blood during arousal. That is why it increases in size when stimulated and presses the vagina during intercourse, favoring that during the penetration, the vagina sensitivity increases. In each woman, the clitoris has a different shape and size. For a long time, it was considered that the length of this organ was about 3 centimeters, but it has been discovered that it reaches up to 10 in some cases. Its function is to give sexual pleasure to the woman and that this, unlike the man, can be multi-orgasmic.

The clitoris is an inexhaustible source of sexual pleasure for women and it is practically impossible for it to reach high levels of arousal or reach orgasm if this erogenous point is neglected. It is she who, in a natural and uninhibited way, must communicate to the lover in what way she enjoys the most since due to her delicacy, too much friction or mechanical movements at this point instead of exciting can end up numbing the area. It is also important to lubricate - with saliva or with the vaginal juice itself - before starting the friction so that the wave of joy increases.

If the woman knows how to guide the lover by teaching him how to enjoy more, by manual or oral stimulation in the clitoris, the frequency and speed with which she wishes to receive it and in what posture it is possible to excite her during penetration, the enjoyment of both will be fuller.

Chapter 2: Sex and Spirituality

The problem with picking and choosing from an ancient text like the Kama Sutra, which is thought to have been compiled in the 2nd century (although it was likely composed somewhere between 400 and 300 BCE), is that for it to mean something you have to take it within the context of the time. In reality, only 20% of the actual Kama Sutra outlined explicit sexual positions and the majority of these that we will focus on were for heteronormative couples (although there are some queer-friendly passages in the text as well as suggestions). The Kama Sutra is compiled as a number of prove and poetic verses and is thought to be attributed to the sage Vatsyayana and most of the text takes into account Indian philosophy and how to live a virtuous life by elaborating on the nature of desire and its effect on our worldly persons.

For our purposes, it's important to analyze our own approach to relationships and love. How do we define love personally? As something physical or intellectual, or both? This, really, is the purpose of the Kama Sutra: to make us think critically and emotionally about our interactions with those we hold dear. In essence, we are trying to achieve a union, and the most direct metaphorical connection to this is the act of sex.

As a physical sort of communion, it is no surprise that it can either bend or break a relationship, and even the Kama Sutra acknowledges that this is something to be aware of. According to their ancient traditions, people were and are guided by energies that inhabit the body – this is not a unique cosmological approach since many societies enculturate the idea of being 'in harmony' with powers or forces that defy the imagination. In the Indian tradition, however, this link between the spiritual and physical is best exemplified by the embodiment of the genitals. In Sanskrit, these were called 'lingam' (for the male reproductive system) and 'yoni' (for the female reproductive system) and were thought to represent the genitals of Shiva and his wife.

Understanding – and not being ashamed – of our genitals, and an appreciation for their uniqueness and for their ability to elicit pleasure in others is a profound and tangible form of happiness. And regarding them (not necessarily as the metaphorical organs of gods, per se) as something sacred is the first step in being able to share the experience of sex with a partner.

How to Get Started:

Before we get too hot and heavy, we want to start slow – sex is not supposed to be a hasty or cathartic act, but something to savor. To this end, foreplay becomes a huge element of the sexual act, helping us to not only become comfortable with our own bodies and the bodies of our lovers but also stimulating physical arousal and fostering a sense of safety and intimacy.

Safety and Security are probably two of the most crucial elements between lovers – if you don't feel safe, if you are stressed or embarrassed, or more importantly if you're afraid of something, then sex can be a stifling and damaging process, and the union we spoke of will not be possible. Let's look at some of the concrete and specific ways we can include foreplay and create a safe space.

1. The Kama Sutra Embrace – this should always be the first thing lovers practice, and involves touching each other; however the word embrace doesn't just mean giving hugs, it means using your entire body to hold another person. Take turns among each other pressing and touching the other on their body, running your fingers along their arms, across their belly, over their chest, and down their legs. The idea here is to physically map

one another's bodies. This helps bring a full *tactile awareness* to the one being touched but is also a good way to help build trust between partners. You can also try kissing one another, or brushing your lips across certain parts of the body – but the key here is gentleness; let your caresses be as soft as flower petals, and let your lover want more than what you're giving.

2. Kissing – the Kama Sutra is quite explicit about how kissing should be, and again gentleness is the key. The slower you are able to kiss, the longer you can draw out the process of foreplay, and the more stimulated both lovers will become. This will also heighten arousal and make the actual act of sex all the more pleasurable. This is also, in a way, a sort of test of patience for both parties, and you are encouraged to seek out parts of the body that aren't normally considered "sexy" – for example, try kissing the inside of the elbow, the top of the scapula, the knee, etc.

3. Using Nails/Biting – varying the sort of tactile stimulus you deliver to your partner is also

emphasized. For example, drawing your nails across their stomach, or allowing yourself to nibble parts of the body. Because the mouth is considered one of the most erogenous parts of the body, it is pleasurable for both people.

Positive Sexual Environments

As mentioned, the Kama Sutra has a lot of chapters designed to elucidate the fact that love is not just a physical act, but also an intellectual and emotional one. While we would like to focus on the physical aspects, being able to develop an environment that is conducive to sexual trust is indispensable. Some suggestions include being able to fill your room with things that both of you love or that you can engage in both before and after – for example, books that you both like, a drawing pad, musical instruments, chess, or other activities that can accompany lovemaking.

It is also important that you both feel comfortable. Creating a 'nest' for yourselves that includes soft blankets, pillows, and fragrant candles can help produce a romantic atmosphere and put you both at ease (especially if you're trying something together for the first time).

Music can also be an aphrodisiac of sorts. But don't worry if you don't play and instrument yourself –

having a soft slow-paced instrumental music playing in the background as you engage in foreplay is another great way to ease both lovers into the moment and help keep you at a gradual pace. Remember again, we're trying to savor the experience of one another, not rush through it!

Aquatic Is A No-No?

Another amusing aspect of the Kama Sutra is that Vatsyayana advocated that the best way to learn the following techniques and sexual positions was to practice them in water. There are some obvious logical reasons for this, especially ones that involve a lot of flexibility or strength (such as holding your lover up while making love, all at the mercy of gravity), and quite frankly we think it's a good idea. That said, Vatsyayana went on to clarify that there was a certain unethical or 'dirtiness' associated with copulating in water that tied in heavily to the spiritual and religious tenor of the day – while some of these taboos and customs may not make much sense today, and you are by no

Chapter 3: Prepare Mind and Body for Sex

Creating the right environment and mood for an intimate massage is as important as the massage itself. Being disturbed halfway through the massage or finding out that you are feeling cold or uncomfortable can spoil the experience.

An abandoned or interrupted intimate massage can have long-term effects on you and put you off from trying it again because you are afraid of being disappointed again. It is therefore important that you take the following preparatory steps to ensure you and your lover enjoy a complete, blissful and fulfilling massage session.

Peace and privacy

Make sure that you will be undisturbed during the massage. This means planning and preparing to eliminate any potential interruptions. The last thing you want is to receive a phone call during the massage. So turn off your phone or put it in silent mode. Make sure the place or room is quiet, peaceful and pleasant, and that it also affords privacy. Lock the door and put a 'Do

Not Disturb' sign if you are in a hotel room. If you are at home, then choose a time that is appropriate when it will be less likely to expect friends or family to come visiting.

The stereotypical ambiance will mean closing the windows and drawing the blinds or curtain closed, dimming the lights and playing some soft music. However, there are no hard and fast rules to do so. You can leave the windows open or the curtains open, if you want to and think that you will still have privacy. You may also prefer silence instead of playing any music.

The lights are also optional. You may dim them or keep them as usual. Some people prefer to light candles or some incense. Talk it over with your lover and choose what you both prefer and feel comfortable with.

Set the temperature on the air conditioner before you begin. Remember that as the body relaxes, the receiver may tend to feel cold, so don't turn the thermostat too low or the fan too high. At the same time, if it is summer and you are in a place that has tropical weather, then be prepared to sweat. Keep some towels and a jug of cool lemonade or water with some glasses nearby and handy.

Feather the nest

More than music or lighting candles, the most important part of preparing for an intimate massage is to choose the place where the receiver will be comfortable. If you are willing to invest in a professional massage table, that's well and good but you don't necessarily have to.

You can lay a mat on the floor and place some clean sheets or a blanket for your lover to lie down. Though some people don't mind using the bed, it's not ideal nor comfortable for various reasons. For instance, you will be using oil during the massage which may stain the mattress. Another very valid reason is that the surface of the bed is not as firm as the floor and this is important for the receiver's comfort.

Clear a place on the floor and arrange everything required; a mat or a thin mattress, some sheets, some blankets, cushions or pillows, towels, oil and anything else you may need.

It's up to you to lubricate or not

Using oil as a lubricant during the massage is optional. Some people may prefer not to use any oil. Not using oil for a full body massage is permissible but it is recommended that you use some kind of lubricant to perform the Yoni massage or the Lingam massage. Since both these massages involve contact with highly sensitive parts such as the vagina, clitoris, penis or testicles, not using oil or lubricant can cause discomfort or even pain.

If you are using oil, then make sure it is suitable for massage. Some of the most commonly preferred massage oils are almond oil, coconut oil or grapeseed oil.

Use oil that is natural and or organic rather than something that is synthetically concocted or blended. It is also a good idea to use oils that you have tried and tested. You don't want any skin irritation, rashes or any form allergic reaction.

Bath or shower

It is recommended that you bathe or shower before a massage to truly enjoy it. It is also healthy and hygienic to do so. A nice slow warm bath before beginning your massage will help relax the muscles and also make the skin feel supple. You may also consider taking a shower together before beginning to set the mood for intimacy.

An intimate massage session has the power to take you to heights of pleasure you've never before experienced. So prepare well to enjoy the pleasure without any limitations or hiccups. In the next two chapters, we look at some of the most intimate ways to pleasure your lover.

These techniques may seem like foreplay because they involve direct contact and massage of your lover's erogenous zones and sexual parts but it is essential to keep in mind that you don't necessarily need to have a goal of sexual intercourse or orgasm.

These intensely pleasurable massage techniques will enable you to experience intense erotic sensations if you are willing to explore them for their own sake and without any prejudice or preconceived expectations. These massages can help you connect not just physically and sexually but emotionally and spiritually as well.

Chapter 4: Keep Your Enemy Closer

Keep your friends close, and your enemies closer. Men rarely talk about premature ejaculation because this is a direct insult to their ego. But as self-help anonymous groups dictate, the first step to solving the problem is admitting you have a problem.

Premature ejaculation is spilling semen way before you or your partner intended. This may happen shortly after penile penetration into the vagina. In some cases, this happens even before penetration is performed. This may cause dissatisfaction to both partners and when no improvement is made, it may certainly be a cause of problems.

Men of all ages are affected by premature ejaculation. Most men, if not all, at one point in their lives, may have gone through this problem. The complaints seem to arise from different situations and there is no definite cause for the condition. It is believed that the cause is multi-factorial.

Some theories say that it is caused by initial overstimulation and lack of control of it. Others say that it may be due to a lack of practice or long periods without intercourse.

Psychological causes may also play a part. This includes experiences of previous trauma and loss of confidence due to frequent experiences of premature ejaculation.

There may also be relational causes, such as less attraction to your partner. A male who also feels inferior to his partner, for whatever reason, may also exhibit these conditions.

Spiritual and social influences may also cause someone of high moral standards to view sex as a sinful activity and cause sexual problems.

The physical aspect of premature ejaculation is the very last to be investigated once all the aforementioned causes have been treated or ruled out. Physical causes of premature ejaculation are rare. Deeper evaluation may reveal problems in the reproductive system or the urinary tract.

With prolonged premature ejaculation, more severe erectile dysfunctions may occur. As with most conditions, early detection is the key. The earlier you set forth to solve the problem, the earlier treatments and solutions can be made.

The important thing you should note is that premature ejaculation is not a life-long condition. It is transient as it is treatable. Through diligence, healthy living, and proper care of your package, you will be able to control the situation.

Treatments and Drugs

Like most things there are certain options for treatment for premature ejaculation. It isn't the end of the world and it doesn't mean that you have any serious medical conditions. Only a very tiny number of people can actually attribute premature ejaculation to a medical complaint but if you are at all uncertain, you should go and see your doctor. Treatment options include topical anesthetics, behavioral techniques, counseling and oral medications. Do keep in mind that the results are not going to be instant, except perhaps in the case of Viagra or other similar medications, and it may take time to find the right treatment for you.

Behavioral Techniques

Therapy may be prescribed and this will involve a number of simple steps for you take, steps like masturbating a couple of hours before you are going to have sex. This can help you to slow down ejaculation during the actual act and help you to last longer. You may also be told that you should avoid actual penetration during sex for a while and concentrate your efforts on other types of sex play. That can help to remove a lot of the pressure from sex as you won't be expected to "perform" as it were.

Pause and Squeeze

This technique is often touted by doctors as a good way of holding things back and it will involve your partner. It works like this:

- You should begin sex as you would normally, making sure your penis is stimulated almost to the point of ejaculation

- At that point, your woman will need to squeeze your penis at the end where the head and shaft join one another. She should hold the squeeze for a few seconds, until you lose the urge to ejaculate

- Once she releases you from the squeeze, wait another 30 seconds then resume your foreplay. You might find that your penis loses some of its rigidity when it is squeezed but don't worry; once you get back down to the pleasure, your erection will return!

- Again, when you get to the point of ejaculation, your partner will squeeze again

This should be repeated as many times as you feel necessary until you get to the stage where you can actually penetrate your partner without immediate ejaculation taking place. After a while of doing this, you will get to grips, if you'll pardon the pun, with knowing how to stop yourself ejaculating straight away and you won't need to continue with this technique

Topical Anesthetic

These are sprays and creams that contain an agent like prilocaine and lidocaine, agents that cause numbing. If your doctor recommends this course of action, you will have to apply the cream or spray a little while before you are going to have sex, so that the sensation is reduced and you can delay your ejaculation. You can purchase these products over the counter but it is best to go to your doctor.

While topical anesthetics can be effective, they do have the potential for side effects. Some users have reported a decrease in sexual pleasure and a loss of sensitivity and, in other cases, the woman has reported feeling the same thing. Also, if you have to apply these creams a short while before you have sex, it means that you are having to plan it and that means the fun is gone, there is no spontaneity anymore.

Oral Medication

There are a few oral medications that can help to slow down an orgasm from happening but many of them are not actually approved by the FDA for the treatment of premature ejaculation. However, that doesn't stop them from being used and include antidepressants, phosphodiesterase-5 inhibitors, and analgesics. These might be prescribed for daily use or to be taken on-demand, and they may also be prescribed as part of a plan that includes other treatments as well.

- Antidepressants – Some men have had great success with using these to delay things a little, simply because one of the side effects of most antidepressants is a delay in orgasm. The most common ones prescribed for this purpose are of the serotonin reuptake inhibitor family – Zoloft, Paxil, Prozac or Sarafem. If these are not successful in helping to slow down the time it takes you to ejaculate, you may well be prescribed Anafranil, or clomipramine – a tricyclic antidepressant. Unfortunately, the possible side effects of nausea, a dry mouth, feeling drowsy and a decrease in libido (not what you want) may be enough to put you off taking this one

- Analgesics – Perhaps the better known of these is Tramadol, normally prescribed as a painkiller with a side effect of delaying ejaculation. It may only be given to you AFTER the above SSRI medication has been tried and failed Again, the side effect may be unpleasant enough to make you not want to take it.

- Phosphodiesterase-5 Inhibitors – These medications are generally used as a way of treating erectile dysfunction but can also help in cases of premature ejaculation and include Viagra, Revatio, Cialis, Adcirca, Staxyn, and Levitra. Side effects may include flushing of the face, headaches, temporary changes to your vision and nasal congestion

Counseling

Also called Talk Therapy, counseling involves you sitting down with a mental health provider and talking about your experiences and your relationships. The idea behind this is that it can help to cut down the amount of anxiety you feel about your performance in bed and to help you cope better with stress. This is normally used in conjunction with drug therapy.

A Personal Story – How I Dealt with Premature Ejaculation

This the story of how one man overcame premature ejaculation; we'll call him Sam for the sake of preserving his identity. Hopefully, his story will help you to see that you too can overcome this troubling situation. It might also go some way towards showing you that, truly, you are not alone. More men than you realize suffer from premature ejaculation; they just don't talk about it, mainly because of the perceived embarrassment and the stress it causes. Without wasting any more time, let's hear what Sam has to say

The loss of my virginity – and my self-respect

Some people say that too much masturbation, rushed masturbation at that, causes premature ejaculation. While this isn't true of everyone, I'm pretty sure that was at least partly to blame for me. When I was a kid, masturbation was very much a taboo subject and, like a lot of guys, I would rush it without giving it any thought.

I can't blame it all on that. I think some of it comes down to when I lost my virginity.

I was a bit of a late starter, not losing my virginity until I reached the age of 19. I met the girl in a nightclub, she was a friend of a friend and, after the nightclub shut we headed back to my place to carry on with the fun we'd been having that night in the club.

Things heated up pretty quickly and, already pretty damn excited from the hours I'd spent dancing close with her, with all the flirting and the foreplay, we never even got close to having sex the first time – I was just too quick. At that point, I didn't know anything about premature ejaculation, had never even heard of it, but I did think that it would have been nicer to have lasted beyond zero seconds!

At the time I didn't realize it but, in that one single moment, my sexual confidence was knocked for six. In the way that many women do, she didn't let on how disappointed she as and, fair play to her, she tried so hard to make me feel that it was OK. Clearly, though, it wasn't.

Sadly, the second time was no better and, at that point, I was embarrassed and horrified, not just for me but for her too. What didn't occur to me was that this was the start of everything, the beginning of all my anxieties over performance.

And, just to add a bit more fuel to the fire, I now realize that my penis is physically sensitive – doomed from the start.

The excuses, the silence

To my shock and amazement, she stayed with me but over the next week or so, I found out how bad the problem really was. If I waited for 24 hours or more between sex sessions, I was done for, I couldn't last longer than a minute at the absolute most. If we had sex over and over again I would get better although I still never really managed to get over the five-minute mark. And that was only if she was prepared to wait for the third or fourth time that was a bit better.

As the months passed, our sexual relations got less and less. Do you know what the most shocking thing is, though? We never once talked about it – ever

To this day, the most embarrassing thing for me is that I never spoke to any partner about this problem over the next few years and I never did anything about it, either. Not even when I finally took the plunge and got married. Perhaps even worse is that none of my partners nor my wife ever mentioned it either. Well, my wife (now my ex-wife) would sometimes call me a "bastard", jokingly when I came too early.

To be fair, we would talk occasionally about the fact that I would come quickly on most occasions but we never talked about it in a way that would register it as a problem that needed to be fixed. All that happened is, like my first girlfriend, the sex got less and less to the point where it was a rare occurrence.

Selfishly, I turned the situation around and said that it happened because we didn't have sex very often and when we did, I just couldn't handle it. Whilst this is, in a small way, true, it doesn't change the fact that I should have sorted this problem sooner, that it was my problem, not hers.

Ironically, after I split up with my ex-wife (not because of the problems with sex), I could finally admit that I had a problem, a serious one that needed dealing with. The day I admitted it is a day I remember more clearly than the day I finally lost my virginity. It was an awful day as well as being a fantastic day. It was awful because, by admitting that I actually had this problem also made me realize that is should have admitted it sooner, many years sooner. I sat there and I thought about all the women I had left frustrated, screaming silently that I couldn't make it last. How many of them told their friends, people that I used to socialize with?

On the good side, the fact that I had finally acknowledged that I had a problem meant I could take steps to solve it.

Taking the first steps

As a man who spent so many years denying that I had a problem, ignoring it, when I finally did admit that is suffered from premature ejaculation, I suddenly found that I was extremely dedicated to solving the problem.

Obviously, the worst and hardest bit was actually admitting that there was a problem. The rest, all the research and the steps in dealing with it, would be easy in comparison, or at least, I hoped they would. The first thing I did was searched the internet and read up on the subject in men's health publications but, sadly, I found most of the information was somewhat vague. Then I discovered a book called The Ejaculation Trainer.

That book was responsible for two things – it gave me hope ad it gave me homework to do. Apparently, the key to unlocking the problem of premature ejaculation is in practicing lots of different techniques while masturbating and/or having sex.

I discovered that there was no instant cure, that these techniques would pay off but not straight away. There were some tips that I could try straight away though and I did.

The next time I was lucky enough to have sex, I tried to use a number of the instant techniques and, yes, there were definitely a few improvements. It was hit and miss, though – sometimes I found I was lasting quite a bit longer while other times it was only a fraction longer.

The time I tried desensitization products

I never even knew these things existed until I read somewhere that you don't need to use them. Well, of course, that got my mind whirring. I already knew that I had a sensitive penis so it was worth a try, wasn't it?

The first one I tried was condoms impregnated with benzocaine – trust me guys, don't bother. Annoying isn't the word here. I tried a product called Priligy, but aside from the fact that it didn't really agree with me, it just didn't work.

I went on to try out a whole load of creams and sprays but, one after the other, they caused me problems or they just didn't work. The more I tried, the more frustrated I became because nothing seemed to work. Then I found a product called Promescent and, by God, it worked. Only as a temporary measure but it was a good one and, to my mind, a miracle.

So now I had this product that was helping me to last for between 10 and 20 minutes at a time, pretty good for the guy who never got past a couple of minutes before. Time to focus on the natural techniques I had learned to see if I could rid myself of this embarrassing and frustrating problem.

Natural techniques

For a couple of months, I stayed away from the women and kept to myself I needed time to get these techniques sorted and put them to the test. I practiced every single day and also learned to understand both my body and how to control my levels of arousal.

It must have been another two months before I was in a position to have sex again and I could put it all to the test. It was very difficult not to feel anxiety but it was important that I didn't. I had already done quite a bit of research about performance anxiety and I was fully prepared in having to deal with it; it seemed that all of the efforts I put in had paid off.

That first time again can't really be counted as a reliable marker because I'm ashamed to say, I was a little drunk, although this wasn't altogether a bad thing – alcohol does help me in that department! The next day when I had sex again was a different matter – I found that I could last much longer than I ever had before.

But, do you know what the most ironic thing about all of this is? I had come to realize that, by talking about it, the anxiety would be reduced and I would be able to last a lot longer. Believe me, the most awesome moment was when the woman I was with, the woman I had told about my problem, looked me in the eye and said, "trust me, you don't have a problem".

Could I at long last, say that I had overcome the problem of premature ejaculation?

It's an ongoing thing

What I came to understand is that, if these natural techniques were going to work forever I had to keep on doing them. If I slack off, my performance times drop, more so when I have been without a partner for a while and stayed away from women.

I have to regularly practice Kegel exercises or my strength starts to go, as does my control. I have to make sure that, whether I am with a partner or on my own, I take my time so I don't end going back to the bad habit of rushing.

If I chuck aside everything I learned about controlling my level of arousal, about breathing properly about learning when to stop, and all the other important things I learned, and just go at it, the difference in performance times just sucks. There is little I can do about it except for keeping up the techniques and the learning.

And, what doesn't help, I still have a sensitive penis; the likelihood is, it will probably always be that way and, I feel it is because of that, when I am with a new partner after being alone for a bit, that I still have problems.

In all honesty, that is when it is the most difficult to get all of the techniques I learned to work. So, when you have been without a partner for a while and you have had issues with premature ejaculation, it is important to be realistic in your expectation of how things are going to be with a new partner, at least to start with.

The best advice I can give you

If it has suddenly occurred to you that you are not lasting as long as you should be in bed, the most important thing that must concentrate on is focusing your efforts on dealing with the problems. Don't do what I did, don't ignore it, the fact that you have a problem because it isn't going away. In fact, it will only get worse.

Do your research, find out exactly what works for you and never give up. The hardest part is n admitting that you have the problem in the first place; the rest, while not plain sailing, is considerably easier to deal with. Trial and error will play a big part in the next few months of your life but you will get there.

Now I can tell you something. I spent many years studying Psychology and I worked in mental health. So, how did it take me so many years to accept that I had a problem, that it was my responsibility and that I needed to deal with it? The point is, it doesn't matter who you are, it doesn't matter what you do as a job or what you study; the important thing is that you learn from my mistakes and don't ignore it,

Three years later

That was three years ago and, I am ecstatic to report, things are getting better by the day. A time has passed, I have learned to fully understand my body and levels of arousal; I can now determine when I get to the point of overheating and in danger of rushing things.

I can exert enough control over myself now to the stage where I can proudly say that I no longer suffer from the problem of premature ejaculation. 10 minutes or more are the norm for me now, on many occasions I can go for much longer.

Things take a step backward if I am in a high state of arousal and I don't use a condom but I now have a confidence I never had before; I can take full control of my sex life and I can do everything I need to keep things in check.

I don't use any kind of delay spray or desensitizing cream and over the years have come to realize that using natural techniques is the only way to deal with this.

Best advice? Don't hold back, get started on learning how you can control yourself today and learn how to last much longer in bed.

Many of the natural and other techniques that Sam used to help him are discussed throughout this book.

Chapter 5: Reconnect With Your Partner

Whether you've been dating for a couple of months or a couple of decades, it's absolutely typical and solid for sexual longing to rhythmic movement over the span of a relationship. However, in the event that the respite has been too yearning for you and/or your accomplice, you may need some assistance in sexually reconnecting once more.

Life gets occupied. Calendars act as a burden. Also, like most types of self-care, our sexual experiences... the very thing that can be topping us off superior to anything whatever else... regularly gets returned on the burner. By sexually reconnecting with your spouse you'll feel more content every day, your contentions will either disseminate or de-raise speedier, and you will feel all the more profoundly associated with your better half all through your relationship. A sound sexual coexistence is one of the significant discussions that you have with your spouse on a continuous premised... and on the off chance that you've basically quit imparting, your relationship is going to take a colossal hit.

Join with your own body first

Keeping in mind the end goal to have a sound sex drive, solid relationship to your sexuality, and general nice sentiments about your body, it's genuinely basic that you feel associated with your own body.

It's inexorably normal, today like never before, to feel separated from our physical bodies. As a general public we tend to practice less, invest less energy in nature, invest additional time on computerized gadgets, and devour more erotic entertainment than at some other point ever. What's more, as an aggregate result, we frequently feel extremely in our heads rather than our bodies. Without that previous extension constructed between our brains to our bodies, it's hard to have a solid moxie and considerably harder to completely appreciate the sexual delight we're encountering as we're encountering it.

Keeping in mind the end goal to balance this excessively 'in our mind' method for living you can do a couple of things.

- Invest energy in nature. Go sit in a woodland (or in a recreation center) with your exposed feet on the ground. Feel the breeze on your body. Breathe in the aroma of your surroundings. Completely drop into the occasion.

- Activity. Go for strolls. Run. Do yoga. Go to the rec center. Do whatever medium-high power game feels the best time/fun-loving/trying for you. The oxygenation and cell reclamation enhances your sexual pleasure and stamina, as well as it equalizations your invulnerable framework and gives your sex drive a jolt.

- Scrub down. Get kneads. Do anything that makes you feel the physical outer sensation that re-sharpens you to how your body encounters touch. Talking about which...

- Masturbation. Every single awesome beau does. Masturbation is one of the best ways you can all the while re-sharpen to your body while likewise recollecting/finding/refining precisely what sort of sexual incitement you locate the most pleasurable. Put aside standard time to see what you appreciate the most while jerking off (paying little heed to regardless of whether you peak) and you'll see the advantages make an interpretation of themselves into your sexual coexistence in a way that you never thought conceivable.

Uproot any significant blocks through discussion

There's unquestionably something to be said in regards to "interface to begin with, impart second." And generally I concur with along these lines of considering. Be that as it may, if your sexual coexistence has been in a respite for some time (and "a while" can mean whatever you need it to mean) there are likely a few things that you or your spouse need to say keeping in mind the end goal to feel like you can sexually reconnect once more. Possibly there's been an uncertain contention that should be tended to. Possibly there are certain stressors that one or both of you have been juggling and you need an open discussion about it. Possibly you simply need to check in with one another and have a genuine, profound discussion.

Whatever arrives that should be tended to, it likely should be tended to before the sexual vitality can begin streaming between you once more (to the extent that you both realize that it can). Whether you have the conversation(s) in or out of the room is dependent upon you. Wherever you feel the most agreeable, that is the place it ought to happen.

Possibly you have to make inquiries like.

"How have you been feeling about our sexual coexistence of late?"

"How have you been feeling about us of late?"

"Is there any uncertain stuff that you feel like we have to discuss?"

Sparkle the notorious light into the dim corners of the majority of the implicit things between you... and you may be astounded in respect to how the all the more profound, fair truth that is called into the light, the more the sexual vitality begins to stream once more. It's not unprecedented for unthinkable themes to be discussed and after that one or both spouses feel a moment shift noticeable all around that leads them to destroy one another with sexual enthusiasm. I sincerely trust that if individuals all the more as often as possible used the strength that it takes to have the intense discussions in their connections, the Viagra/Cialis/Levitra/E.D. pills business sector would lose 20% of their income overnight. The speediest path to a stone hard erection or a smooth, wet vagina may simply be a genuine, soul exposing discussion about something genuine.

More truth = more sexual stream = more capacity to sexually connect.

Begin with these association works out

Since the significant points have been verbally tended to and managed in a cherishing, empathetic way, we can get to the more physical association works out.

I have found that, for me by and by and for endless customers, these taking after association activities are super effective for helping us moderate down, drop into the occasion, furthermore, reconnect with our spouse in a way that we aren't inclined to doing all the time (unless you've been tailing me for some time and consistently utilize my tips).

7 breath brow association

I have expounded on this one in the past in my article 6 Association Practices For Couples, and it bears rehashing. It's straightforward. You gradually meet up, brow to temple (or third eye to third eye for you all the more profoundly slanted people), and you experience seven rounds of associated breaths. You breathe in gradually together, and breathe out gradually together at least seven times. You do this without talking, and with your eyes shut. This activity helps you truly match up to your accomplice, and it additionally energizes you both to back off and concentrate on your breath. It's a superb activity to use to pick up a clear, moderate snippet of association regardless of what the setting is. I have a few hitched customers who do this activity with their spouse each morning and consistently, as their non-debatable non-verbal check-in.

Nestle for 10+ minutes

Nestling is fabulous. One of the best things that we can accomplish for our sexual association is re-coordinate more touch into our lives. Also, one of the most ideal ways we can do that most proficiently? Rather than flipping through Instagram, checking our email, or perusing our computerized books before we nap off, why not take a stab at organizing developed nestle sessions?

As people, we all ache for touch... and we particularly cherish it from individuals that we as of now love also, worship. So stop your gadgets, set a clock on the off chance that you need to, and snuggle for some time. The cheerful chemicals that get discharged in your cerebrum will help you rest superior to very nearly whatever else you can do before bed at any rate.

Kiss for 10+ minutes

Keep in mind when you were more youthful and kissing was its own prize, and not only a preparatory step that unavoidably prompt sex (as is basic in long haul connections)? All things considered, prepare to have your mind blown. Kissing is still generally as magnificent.

Kissing is a profoundly cozy act, however we regularly hurry through it too rapidly to recollect that fundamental certainty. Investigate your accomplice's mouth with yours. Grasp their face. Moderate down and completely appreciate that it is so magnificent to kiss somebody you cherish so profoundly. Kissing is a discussion... and it's one that you would prefer not to race through. Certainly. Some touching/grabbing/pounding may normally happen in your 10+ moment make-out session and that is absolutely fine... yet let the kissing become the dominant focal point for some time. You may be amazed in respect to how it's advantages penetrate all through the greater part of your sexual play.

Amplified one-way foreplay

Presently, I don't even truly trust in the word foreplay in light of the fact that it sets up the thought that there is stuff that you do "before sexual play" and afterward the gathered "well done," otherwise known as penetrative sex. I feel that the word sets up an awful outlook for our sexual experiences. In any case, it's still a typical word so I'll meet society where it's at. Much the same as backing off and getting a charge out of kissing is incredibly fun (and profoundly close), having non-hurried amplified, one-way foreplay is likewise fun and profoundly imply. I would even contend that foreplay, in the customary comprehension of the word, is the closest part about sex.

We back off and set aside an ideal opportunity to center the total of our consideration on making our spouse feel as well as can be expected potentially feel… through the utilization of our hands, mouths, toys, and whatever else that we can consider/they approach us for. This is likewise where the last point in segment #1 becomes possibly the most important factor… if our spouses have ventured up the allegorical bat when it went to their own particular self-pleasuring, ideally they'll be sufficiently brave to request precisely what they have to feel the best. Furthermore, if they aren't open to asking, we can either ask them straightforwardly amid the sexual play, on the other hand essentially go off of their non-verbal signals (pacing of breath, development of their body, groaning, and so on.).

Whatever you end up doing in your sexual play, moderate down, take as much time as is needed, have a good time what's more, your spouse's joy completely, and alternate so that you each get the opportunity to concentrate on both the giving and the getting stages.

Ruining sessions

Ruining sessions are as basic as their name infers. You and your spouse alternate gifting one another with a continuous piece of time (30 minutes, 60 minutes, three hours... it's dependent upon you) where you extend your physical and sexual closeness (as coordinated by the beneficiary). It's essentially an activity where you at the same time work on being narrow-minded, while additionally expressly requesting what you need.

Possibly your spouse needs you to begin off with a back rub... or kissing, or snuggling. Possibly they need you to go down on them in a sure position for some time. Possibly they need to have moderate, erotic sex with you while you listen to their most loved music coming through noisy, bass-y speakers. Whatever you do amid your ruining sessions is up to the beneficiary (clearly inside of whatever limits you are both alright with).

Keep in mind, this activity is a safe place stretch for many people (particularly the first or two times that you do it) on the grounds that we're not used to expressly inquiring about what we need in bed. So be understanding and adoring with yourself. It's an activity. It will bring about development (in you exclusively and in your relationship). So set aside your time with it, and give it a couple tries (each) before you choose how you feel about it. In the event that you stick with it, it could transform into the best thing that ever happened to your relationship.

Organize it to keep the energy going

While transient blasts 'DO' convey worth to our connections/sexual experiences (like the burst of bliss/association that you get from setting off to a weekend workshop or experimenting with a ruining session one time), they are still only devices. The way that we genuinely and profoundly shift the nature of our connections (and lives as a rule) is by building new propensities.

Whatever you have found has worked the best for you (from kissing to snuggling to ruining sessions and past) out of the above rundown, talk it over with your accomplice, and make a responsibility to make these propensities a piece of your normal schedule.

Placed them in your calendar. Make your association time non-negotiable. I would suggest a supreme least of once every week (in the event that its different hours long) as far as possible up to each morning and/or night. Nothing matters more than the association you feel with your close accomplice. Such a large amount of your bliss, wellbeing, and professional fulfillment is attached to how cheerful you feel in your home life. So make it need number one and see what happens.

A few individuals believe that putting association/discussion/sex/your relationship in your timetable is un-hot - yet I feel that there's nothing sexier.

What's sexier than demonstrating your spouse "I think about you so much that I need you to take up different time-spaces in my date-book... on the grounds that you're justified, despite all the trouble. We're justified, despite all the trouble. Our association is my most noteworthy need in life."

Our time and consideration are the most profitable assets that we will ever have. So give them unreservedly to your spouse and your whole life will thrive. Furthermore, there's nothing sexier than deliberateness.

Chapter 6: Breathing and Diaphragmatic Breathing

Who doesn't love a good orgasm? There's nothing quite like it. We all seek them out and when we find them, are lost to world - briefly. That said, the other type of orgasm – cosmic, rolling and long-lasting – implicates all that we are and for extended periods of time. There is only one way to arrive at this state of bliss and that is through the pursuit of sexual continence. While this may not be for everyone, it's certainly worth a look. Most of us, I'm sure, will be content with re-lighting the flame of passion with our beloved partners. Some of us, though, once that's occurred, will want to take that passion to the next level, which is more intensely spiritual than any other we've discussed. This level of union is the purest form of worship that can be engaged in. Two bodies joined in sexual union, which doesn't have orgasm as its goal, are experiencing a rare state of extended and limitless bliss few others can attain to. For that reason, I'm including this section on supportive exercises for those of you interested in exploring sexual continence and giving it a place in your sacred sexual practice.

Breathing

Improper breathing represents a disconnect between our bodies and our minds. That's because breathing is something we don't think about. It's an automatic, physical function that we do even in the deepest levels of sleep. Breathing mindfully connects our bodies with our minds and opens our awareness to physical sensation. During sexual encounters, particularly when we're seeking to delay orgasm in the service of reaching toward the divine, breathing is a way for us to control the effect of sensation on our orgasmic potential.

There are two principle methods of breathing that can be helpful in this respect. The first is breathing through the nose. Slow, calm breathing, inhaling and exhaling exclusively through the nostrils, is capable of producing a calm, meditative state and sharpening our intellectual connection with the senses, as we experience them. Your metabolic rate, when using this type of breathing, will also be slowed down.

Breathing through the mouth is a natural way of breathing and usually occurs when our bodies demand more oxygen, or when we're expressing an emotion like surprise, or even sorrow. You'll note that when people cry, the mouth is usually open, especially when crying descends into sobbing.

Breathing slowly and mindfully, exhaling and inhaling only through the mouth, also helps the body to release accumulated toxins and helps to relieve tension in the nervous system. Slowing the breathing allows for the body and mind to be integrated into purpose. By briefly holding the breath following inhalation, consciousness is expanded to encompass sensation.

These two basic types of breathing should be practiced with an eye to making them seem more natural. In this way, employing them as part of your sacred sexual ritual will be less forced and much more part of what you're living as you enjoy your partner in divine sexual union. Perfecting these before trying the technique I'm about to describe to you is highly recommended.

Breathing deeply is also a way of reducing the influence of stress in your life. As most of us have figured out, stress can put a damper on sex. If we're so exhausted by the endless challenges of everyday living, by the time we've come home to our beloved, how are we to even think about engaging in satisfying, transcendent sex? Getting the stress in our lives under control should be part of our breathing practice and one of the many benefits intentionally-practiced breathing offers.

During sex, depending on your level of mastery over your breathing, the most important thing you can do is to be aware of how you're breathing. Shallow or sharp breaths in the heat of the moment may be unavoidable, to a point. But if you're practicing sexual continence, then it's important both partners be fully aware of the quality of their breathing. Monitoring it and ensuring that your breathing is even and slow helps keep your body relaxed. It also ensures that oxygen is being delivered efficiently and filling your blood cells. This keeps you alive to the moment and focused on what you're doing, which assists you to engage the fullness of your sensuality in your ritual sexual practice.

Re-birthing breathing

This technique's intent is to take us back to the first breath we ever drew – the one directly following our arrival on earth. By returning us to that moment, we can experience ourselves on an entirely different level, much more in tune with the cosmos. This method is part of re-connecting with ourselves at the very deepest level.

Lying on your back, with your mouth open, begin to breathe through the mouth, slowly and naturally. Don't force yourself to breathe in any particular way. Just open your mouth and intentionally inhale and exhale through it. Now fill your lungs with air by slowly inhaling. When you're ready to exhale, you'll feel your abdomen deflating naturally.

As you're performing this breathing exercise, think of breathing with your entire body. Intellectually connect those areas of your body you don't normally associate with breathing into the action of your exhalations and inhalations. Visualize your entire body being filled with air, as you slowly inhale and exhale. You will, if you proceed with consistency, take note of a variety of sensations in your body, including tingling. These are due to the influx of oxygen into your system provoked by slow and steady breathing. You will also notice, as you proceed, that your breathing gradually slows even further. You may sense that you are drifting into a somewhat altered state of consciousness (at least, I hope you do).

It's in this altered state, that you'll be able to experience your body and mind from another perspective. You may find that you're able to visualize yourself in the womb, or in another place from the one you're in (astral projection). What you experience with this exercise is the nature of the universe itself, which is a state of tension holding it together. The tension between opposites (as expressed in the co-creative, sacred sex act) is the glue in the universal structure and is also expressed as the simultaneous expansion and contraction of all that is. This is embodied in your breathing. By fully (but naturally) expelling the air from your lungs in this breathing technique, you are both calling on the past (which is present) and pushing it from you, as you breathe. As you pull air into your lungs, you are pulling the change you desire to know in yourself, inside you, distributing it throughout your body. This plays out as a means of becoming the arya you seek to be.

As you breathe, your intellect and your body will work together to identify points at which you've become blocked, or stuck. This will allow you the opportunity to address these threats to your continuing growth. You may also, with practice, arrive at the point at which you perceive absolutely nothing, and have no discernible thoughts and no consciousness. This is the most desired state achievable, using the re-birthing breathing exercise – that of non-being. Only in this state is a true revelation of the self possible, for just beyond it is a place that represents the boundary between our perceptions of life and reality and the truth. That truth is something completely "other"; something that we can't experience in consciousness. In reaching this place, the ecstasy of the truth will open the door to your deepest self-revelation and profound changes that will continue to affect you, long after the breathing exercise has been completed. You will take those changes into the practice of your sacred sexuality and share them with your partner.

In Kama Sutra, sex partners share with one another a divine experience of give and take. This reciprocity should, of course, extend to these breathing exercises. Your partner should also be practicing them.

Chapter 7: Setting the Mood

Creating the right environment and mood for an intimate massage is as important as the massage itself. Being disturbed halfway through the massage or finding out that you are feeling cold or uncomfortable can spoil the experience.

An abandoned or interrupted intimate massage can have long-term effects on you and put you off from trying it again because you are afraid of being disappointed again. It is therefore important that you take the following preparatory steps to ensure you and your lover enjoy a complete, blissful and fulfilling massage session.

Peace and privacy

Make sure that you will be undisturbed during the massage. This means planning and preparing to eliminate any potential interruptions. The last thing you want is to receive a phone call during the massage. So turn off your phone or put it in silent mode. Make sure the place or room is quiet, peaceful and pleasant, and that it also affords privacy. Lock the door and put a 'Do Not Disturb' sign if you are in a hotel room. If you are at home, then choose a time that is appropriate when it will be less likely to expect friends or family to come visiting.

The stereotypical ambiance will mean closing the windows and drawing the blinds or curtain closed, dimming the lights and playing some soft music. However, there are no hard and fast rules to do so. You can leave the windows open or the curtains open, if you want to and think that you will still have privacy. You may also prefer silence instead of playing any music.

The lights are also optional. You may dim them or keep them as usual. Some people prefer to light candles or some incense. Talk it over with your lover and choose what you both prefer and feel comfortable with.

Set the temperature on the air conditioner before you begin. Remember that as the body relaxes, the receiver may tend to feel cold, so don't turn the thermostat too low or the fan too high. At the same time, if it is summer and you are in a place that has tropical weather, then be prepared to sweat. Keep some towels and a jug of cool lemonade or water with some glasses nearby and handy.

Feather the nest

More than music or lighting candles, the most important part of preparing for an intimate massage is to choose the place where the receiver will be comfortable. If you are willing to invest in a professional massage table, that's well and good but you don't necessarily have to.

You can lay a mat on the floor and place some clean sheets or a blanket for your lover to lie down. Though some people don't mind using the bed, it's not ideal nor comfortable for various reasons. For instance, you will be using oil during the massage which may stain the mattress. Another very valid reason is that the surface of the bed is not as firm as the floor and this is important for the receiver's comfort.

Clear a place on the floor and arrange everything required; a mat or a thin mattress, some sheets, some blankets, cushions or pillows, towels, oil and anything else you may need.

It's up to you to lubricate or not

Using oil as a lubricant during the massage is optional. Some people may prefer not to use any oil. Not using oil for a full body massage is permissible but it is recommended that you use some kind of lubricant to perform the Yoni massage or the Lingam massage. Since both these massages involve contact with highly sensitive parts such as the vagina, clitoris, penis or testicles, not using oil or lubricant can cause discomfort or even pain.

If you are using oil, then make sure it is suitable for massage. Some of the most commonly preferred massage oils are almond oil, coconut oil or grape seed oil.

Use oil that is natural and or organic rather than something that is synthetically concocted or blended. It is also a good idea to use oils that you have tried and tested. You don't want any skin irritation, rashes or any form allergic reaction.

Bath or shower

It is recommended that you bathe or shower before a massage to truly enjoy it. It is also healthy and hygienic to do so. A nice slow warm bath before beginning your massage will help relax the muscles and also make the skin feel supple. You may also consider taking a shower together before beginning to set the mood for intimacy.

An intimate massage session has the power to take you to heights of pleasure you've never before experienced. So prepare well to enjoy the pleasure without any limitations or hiccups. In the next two chapters, we look at some of the most intimate ways to pleasure your lover.

These techniques may seem like foreplay because they involve direct contact and massage of your lover's erogenous zones and sexual parts but it is essential to keep in mind that you don't necessarily need to have a goal of sexual intercourse or orgasm.

These intensely pleasurable massage techniques will enable you to experience intense erotic sensations if you are willing to explore them for their own sake and without any prejudice or preconceived expectations. These massages can help you connect not just physically and sexually but emotionally and spiritually as well.

Chapter 8: Spin Your Chakras and Breathe To Ecstasy

There are many practices that you will come across in this book. These practices are fun and you may find them fascinating! These practices include different sounds, symbols and sights that will help you on your journey to ecstasy. You will learn a few techniques in this chapter. You will need to practice these techniques in order to perfect them. The most important aspect of tantric sex is what you are doing this very second: breathing. It is very important that you breathe properly in order to ensure that you are able to attain the deepest level of intimacy and the highest level of bliss.

Focus on the source of your breath

Have you identified that there is a place in your body where your breathing starts? Do you think it is from your throat or chest or stomach area? It is not supposed to come from either of those areas. You have to make the effort to ensure that you breathe from deep within your body. To ensure that you breathe properly, you will have to take a deep breath. Take the breath in slowly and trace the place where the breathing stops with your hand. Then exhale. The next time you breathe you will have to ensure that you take your breath from as low as your genitals. This helps in firing up the energy that you need to have during sex.

Egg to Eagle

This is a great technique to use when you are sitting. You will have to bend into the shape of a ball. When you are bending you have to exhale swiftly. Bring your hands close to your body and place them on the back of your head. Do you feel your back stretching? Inhale and move up slowly into your sitting position. Stretch your hands as far back as you can. Ensure that your elbows are behind you. You should now feel your chest stretching. Arch your back and throw your chest out. You will now feel all the air rushing into your chest. Continue this exercise. You will be able to breathe well after a few repetitions.

The Wells

The aim of this exercise is to take air into your lungs. You will have to take a lot of air into your lungs. This can only be done when you think of your lungs as wells. You will be able to increase the virtual capacity of your lungs. Keep your arms to your side. After you have inhaled, hold the air for a few seconds and blow all the air out with immense force. It should sound like a gust of wind. Then suck in the air by making as much noise as possible. You will make such sound while making love to your partner. Through this exercise, you will be able to ensure that the sounds you make during sexual intercourse are intense!

Chapter 9: Sexual Domination and Submission

BDSM stands for Bondage and Discipline, Dominance and Submission, and Sadism and Masochism. It is also commonly referred to as kink. Let's take a moment to look at what each of these elements stands for.

Bondage and Discipline

This element refers to the restraint and behavior modification of the submissive. Restraining the submissive can be done in many ways and can range for simple ways such a being tied or handcuffed to the bedpost to advanced techniques such as Shibari, which is a Japanese rope form of bondage. Ceiling hooks and bondage cages can also be used. The discipline part of this involves correcting the sub missive's actions with punishments that can be physical and psychological techniques like spanking or erotic humiliation.

Dominant and Submissive

A BDSM relationship comprises of two components: dominance and submission. Therefore, one person plays the role of the dominant and the other, the submissive. The dominant is responsible for dominating the submissive while the submissive gives up control in a BDSM relationship to the dominant.

Sadism and Masochism

This element of the BDSM involves the giving and receiving of pain. The masochist is the one inflicting the pain and experiences pleasure from doing do. The sadist receives the pain and gets satisfaction from it. Sadism and masochism and dominance and submission differ because the former is about inflicting pain while the latter is about control. These two elements are often present at the same time in a BDSM relationship, but they are not mutually exclusive.

Finding a Balance of Dominance and Submission

People who incorporate BDSM into the sex life of their relationship introduce a power play where one person identifies as the dominant and the other as the submissive. As it refers to BDSM, when the male takes the dominant role, this is called male dominance or maledom. Because the word dominant has a masculine connotation, we often associate the role of dominant as one for men. However, there are women with powerful personalities that can handle being the dominant in the relationship. A dominant female is usually called a dominatrix, and she takes the dominant role in BDSM activities.

Sometimes a person acts as a switch, which is someone that can move between both roles. Activities that are common in BDSM relationships include:

- ____Hair pulling
- ____Fantasy and role-playing
- ____Aggressive language
- Spanking
- Flogging
- Fetishes
- ____Voyeurism and exhibitionism
- Biting
- ____Using a blindfold.
- ____Incorporating candle wax.
- ____Incorporating titles like "Sir" and "Madam"
- ____Group sex

Couples can engage in just one of these activities or a combination, and the level of kink can range from mild to extreme.

When the term BDSM comes up, most people associate it with Fifty Shades of Grey and Rihanna's song about whips and chains. There is much more to this lifestyle choice, however. There is a lot of misinformation around what BDSM is and what it entails. This is mostly due to the betrayal by the media, where it is mostly shown to be some kind of deviant activity that people with a list of psychologies partake in. This is not the case. BDSM is not a good word for physical violence through sexual means. Most of the time, BDSM is associated with general sadism, being mean, and aggressive behavior. If that is what the couple is into, then that is great, but a healthy BDSM relationship does not automatically operate on this premise.

People from all walks of life practice BDSM, and most of them live quite normal lives. That is because they aim of a healthy BDSM relationship is so that both partners are able to please each other and to cater to their individual kinks. The key to living a healthy and happy BDSM lifestyle is to find a balance between domination and submission. A skillful, caring dominant requires having confidence and being sensitive to your partner's needs. You are not just the dominant because you use a strong tone of voice or derogatory language. While the dominant is in a position of control, it is truly the submissive that has the power because the role of the dominant is to cater to the needs of the submissive. The submissive is the one who sets the boundaries and has ultimate control of what happens in the sexual relationship. It may be that the person enjoys sadism under careful infliction of pain. This does not mean uninvited physical abuse, however. A dominant is someone who is very generous because he sees to servicing his or her submissive desires. A good dominant also places a lot of attention on aftercare, which is the time and attention he or she gives to his partner after an intense sexual experience to ensure that the submissive feels cared for and appreciated. Great aftercare activities include cuddling and conversation about what happened and how the submissive feels about it.

BDSM Misconceptions and Stereotypes

There is a lot of information surrounding this kind of sexual lifestyle, and this section is aimed at helping separate fact from fiction. Here are a few stereotypes about kink and information about whether or not they are true.

- *You need fancy equipment to practice a true BDSM lifestyle.* When a lot of people think of BDSM, they think dominatrix in five-inch heels, a flogger, and Andrew's cross behind her, but practicing does not have to be complicated, nor does it require you to buy any special tools. All you need is your imagination and a partner who is just as interested and eager as you to explore BDSM.

- _____*People who practice BDSM only have rough sex.* Rough sex is something that many women and men fantasize about but only have the courage to explore with a partner that they trust to care for them and to ensure their safety as well as their pleasure. If that is what the couple enjoys doing, then more power to them, but BDSM does not automatically translate into extreme or rough play. Sometimes, BDSM to a couple means that one partner is more in charge of making decisions in the bedroom.

Introducing BDSM into a Relationship

Most people are afraid to bring up their BDSM fantasies to someone else. Again, this is likely because of the stigma and taboo connotation that society and families have placed around the subject of domination and submission. However, only a strong, well-founded relationship will survive introducing BDSM elements into it. If you and your partner have built a strong foundation based on trust and consideration, you should be able to openly communicate about your fantasies and the possibility of exploring and reenacting them with that person. Make a list of the things that you would like to experience and talk to your partner about them. Find a neutral location to do this so that your partner does not feel pressured to give you a particular response after your disclosure. If your partner is not very familiar with BDSM, introduce the topic in a way that incites curiosity and promotes positivity toward the subject.

To introduce BDSM into a relationship, start small and work your way up to more extreme elements. Small steps can include watching a BDSM movie together, simple role-playing, or introducing a light spank here and there during love making. Try one activity at a time rather than trying to indulge in everything at once. Always remember to respect each other's boundaries and to keep an open field for negotiations. After you two have indulged in an element of BDSM, remember to check in with each other to ensure that you are both still on the same page and to find out what your partner thinks about the experience.

The important thing to remember is that nobody should feel pressured or coerced into doing anything they do not want to do. Both of you should be open to the ideas and approach them with an adventurous spirit rather than a defensive one.

BDSM for Beginners

Getting kinky with your partner has a lot of benefits, but you two can only enjoy these benefits if you begin with a conversation. Both of you need to be educated about what you are doing and the consequences. Communication is vital in establishing dominant and submissive roles and the limits that each person has in participating in this type of sex. Everything that will happen needs to be consented to prior. You do not want to harm your partner or trigger any psychological consequences. BDSM can be a deeply moving and emotional experience for some people, and mental and emotional health needs to be catered to in addition to physical health. The core components of a successful, long-standing kinky relationship are communication, understanding, trust, and patience. Practicing BDSM is different for every couple. Therefore, stop trying to find a stereotypical example to follow. Go with what feels right to you and your partner. Test the waters and keep what feels right and discard what feels wrong.

With that being said, here are a few general rules that you can use to keep your kink safe as well as pleasurable.

Use a Safe Word

A safeword is a word that a submissive uses to let the dominant know if he should stop, proceed, or slow down the action that he is taking. Some elements of BDSM may involve resistance and restraint. This is the only case where "no" might not really mean "no." Therefore, a safe word allows the dominant to know exactly what his or her submissive is feeling at that moment and how he or she should proceed.

Set Hard Limits

Hard limits are activities that submissive or dominant are dead set against doing. Once your partner has disclosed this hard limit to you, you should never, ever venture into that territory as this spells a lack of concern, care, and consideration. By doing this, you can introduce distrust into your relationship.

Ensure That All Pain Inflicted Is Pleasurable

Some people find pleasure in pain, and this is why spanking and slapping are such popular BDSM activities. However, this should be approached carefully so that the pain remains pleasurable and so that it does not introduce long-term or serious damage to tissue or nerves. There is an art to inflicting the right type of pain in a BDSM relationship, and both parties should be educated and informed before indulging.

Practice Aftercare

Sometimes, some people, especially women, experience a condition known as postcoital dysphoria after sex even of the non-kinky variety. This condition includes symptoms like anxiety, irritability, and motiveless crying. This is a common display in submissive as well, and the dominant should cater to this and provide aftercare in the form of emotional intimacy and communication.

How to Tell If You Are a Dominant, Submissive, or Switch

Determining your role in a BDSM relationship is important as it affects the structure of the relationship and how both parties act and react to BDSM stimuli. The dominant is also sometimes called the top and the submissive, the bottom.

Some people think that this is easy to determine based on a person's personality; however, it is not so cut-and-dry. Some people who are outwardly shy and submissive outside the bedroom find the most pleasure in being the dominant in a sexual relationship, while the opposite may be true for people with flamboyant and dominant personalities outside the bedroom. Some people find out they prefer to be submissive in a sexual relationship simply because they are used to wielding so much control outside of that relationship. They would like to turn the reins over to someone else in the safety of that personal relationship and enjoy being controlled. There is a huge sense of relief that comes with knowing what they are responsible for and what other people are responsible for. This person would like to be taken care of and would like to stop worrying at the moment.

The opposite can also be true. Some people who feel that they do not wield enough control in their everyday life such as their work-life find solace in being dominant in sexual relationships. They would like the satisfaction of having someone else's needs and wants placed in their care and to extend on that satisfaction by catering to those needs and wants in the right way.

There is a more special formula for finding out if you are a dominant, submissive, or switch in a relationship. Some people know instinctively which role they will fulfill, but for others, it is not so easy, and the only way that can be determined is by experimentation and experience. Some people try both roles and realize that they are a lot more comfortable in one, while some people realize that they could switch easily between two based on the session or with the partner. Whatever role that you find most comfort in, know that there is no right or wrong. Do not try to put yourself in a box or label yourself as something you think you should be. The beauty of BDSM is that it gives both you and your partner the chance to explore different dimensions in life because BDSM can extend outside of the bedroom and into other elements of a couple's life. It allows both parties to explore their fantasies in a safe and trusting environment. This can only strengthen the connection between the two parties and, as a result, their relationship.

To help make it easier for you to find out which of these categories you may fall into, here are a few personality traits that each of these persons usually exhibits.

Chapter 10: Reel Life to Real Life

Sex sells. That's a fact that some (or many) may not be comfortable with. You can see it everywhere – magazines, TV, advertisements, and movies. While this move contributes to the corruption of minors, it also benefits those in a relationship since it may stir the fire between them.

Majority of films have love scenes where two people engage in coitus. With the proliferation of nudity in media (think Game of Thrones, Californication, and Lady Gaga), couples have been making more excuses to get turned on and make love. Sex scenes in movies and TV also give them another reason (and inspiration) to up the ante in the bedroom.

Stairway to Heaven

Probably two of the most revised movie scenes that involved a staircase were that of A History of Violence and The Thomas Crown Affair. While the sex seemed so good, one may balk a little after realizing how difficult it is to make love on such an uneven and hard surface. But it is possible—and great.

First of all, this sexual position is not limited to the stairs in your home or in the office building (if you're feeling adventurous). This can also be done in the pool if it has stairs built (which is quite common, anyway). Of course, make sure you have the pool all to yourselves or else you risk someone making a sex video of your escapade—or worse, your grandmother walking in on you.

To do the deed, the woman should be sitting on the stair that is aligned to the man's pelvis whose feet are on the floor and his body leaning towards the girl. This is probably on the second or third step. While sitting, the woman moves her arms back and places them on the stair right behind them. This is important for support. She then spreads her legs as the guy leans over to enter her. The man will need his hands for support but if he's strong enough, he can use one free hand to explore the girl's body adding to the sensation. Make the thrusts deep and wild to help her reach orgasm. If you're in a pool, the thrusting motion creates small waves that may help stimulate the girl.

Backstairs Boogaloo

The Backstairs Boogaloo is another sex position that involves a staircase. The girl positions herself fronting the stairs. Her knees are firmly planted on one step while her hands placed on another to keep her balance. The man then kneels on another step below the girl. He then proceeds to take her from behind. Having both knees on the hard stairs may be uncomfortable so some kind of padding may be necessary. Although with the carnal delight brought about by this position and the risk of getting caught (if you're doing the deed in a public staircase), there might be no time to worry about such things. The man may find it easier to thrust with one leg extended down or one knee bent up. For the woman, leaning her chest closer to the stairs may also make things more comfortable.

The Tabletop Position

One of the sexiest scenes in the Richard Gere and Julia Roberts starred Pretty Woman was their characters' sexual tryst on top of a grand piano. The sexual position in question here does not necessarily need a grand piano (though it does add some much-needed elegance and kinkiness). Any high enough surface may suffice as long as both pelvises can be aligned. It's better if the surface is as high as the waist. The dining table, kitchen counter, washing machine, and the boss' office desk are just a few of the things that come to mind.

The Tabletop Position, also known as the Torrid Tabletop, starts off with the woman sitting with her buttocks at the edge of the high surface. In the said movie's case, Vivian Ward was on top of a grand piano in the dark hotel lounge. The guy then grabs both legs in each arm to spread them. She can also open her legs wide by herself to keep the level of seduction on a high. He then positions himself between her legs. Still standing, he then penetrates the woman's vagina and starts thrusting. The lady can lean back and place her hands on the surface. Leaning her head back can also add to her excitement as she cannot see what is happening. She can only focus on the delectable feeling of having sex. The same can be said when she lies down on her back. As for her legs, she can either let them hang loose or wrap them around the guy. The latter is a good way to have more physical contact.

Speaking of physical contact, she can also lean her body forward to be closer to her man. Embracing him or wrapping her arms around his neck is also a good variation of the Tabletop because of the intimacy it promotes. With her legs locked behind her man and her arms on his neck, he can easily carry her from the table and bring her to the bedroom, all while he's still inside her. They can also move on to the Leg Lock position which basically involves him carrying the girl and thrusting into her without the benefit of a table or any sturdy surface.

Another variation of the Tabletop is the Lying Down Scissors. This is basically the same as the Tabletop. The only difference is her legs are extended up parallel to the guy and crisscrossed with one leg over the other. In other words, the left leg is sitting on his right shoulder while her right leg is on his left shoulder. This position creates more clitoral stimulation because of the tighter feel. This is an enjoyable position for both parties.

The Sneak-A-Peek is another position that is derived or started from the Tabletop Position. This time the woman's butt is hanging from the edge and her forearms flat on the surface behind her for support. The guy holds her feet and places them on his shoulders. This position requires upper body strength as the guy has to carry and support the woman. The best part of the Sneak-A-Peak is the guy can actually see everything from where he is – her face, her breasts, her body, and especially her vagina.

This sexual position is a great way to improve any couple's sex life. The simple fact of using other places other than the bed for sex is a surefire way to make things a tad more exciting than usual. The Tabletop Position can be done anywhere in the house as long as the surface is waist-high. For those who want to go to the extreme, the Tabletop is also the perfect position to do in the office, school or any other public place. As long as both parties are good to go and the place is safe enough that you won't get caught (especially if you don't want to spend the rest of the day convincing your boss not to fire you or your local librarian not to terminate your library card), then this position is something you should always have in your repertoire. Where there's a table, there's always a way to have fun and rather dangerous sex.

Chapter 11: Personal Lubricants

Here's where you're going to spend a few bucks, my friends and yes, it's worth every penny. The return on investment for these goodies is about as high a yield you'll get for any investment you'll ever make. And remember what you're investing in – your relationship and re-discovering the passion you've had with your partner in the past. Your love is worth it and your sex life, with the help of a little slippery fun, will be that much more joyous and thrilling.

We've talked about the usefulness of additional lubrication. I know a lot of people will think it's not necessary, or that there are household items which can just as easily be used, but that's not necessarily the case. Don't forget that you have to wash those sheets, towels, the rug, the curtains, the silk boxers and anything else lube comes into contact with. But part of the fun of lubrication is the fact that you have to go out, select and buy it and that such selection and purchase amounts to a pre-meditation of your mutual pleasure. What could possibly be sexier than going shopping together to find just the right lube? A shopping expedition a deux, followed by a private product demonstration. What fun! Let's talk about some of the various types of lube and what they're best suited to.

Slippin' and a slidin' – the lubrication basics

There are so many activities that lube can make better. Any kind of sex act is rendered much more sexual by the simple act of doing it with lube. So what if you don't need it? More is more! This is sex, people and you want it to be as sensual and lascivious, as slippery and as slidey as you can possibly make it. Being conservative about sex is a bit of a contradiction in terms, if you ask me. Go for the gusto!

Like a machine, when various body parts rub together, friction may occur which inhibits the optimum operation of the machinery involved. To keep everything ticking along seamlessly and without operational breakdown, machines often need to be properly oiled. Human beings have similar needs.

While the human body creates its own versions of sexual lubrication (in the uncircumcised penis and in the vagina, when aroused), sometimes, we want a little more of it. Or perhaps, we'd like some lubrication where it's not naturally produced. There are different kinds of lube and this is the first and most aspect of personal lubricants we're going to discuss, sub-genres not excepted.

Water-based

Most people prefer lubricants that are water-based for good reason – they're easier to clean up after. Getting water-based lube on your sheets isn't a catastrophe. Just throw that mess in the wash and be done with it! Same for your body – this type of lubricant washes off easily.

Water-based lubricants are also kind to the skin, as the water used in them is purified. Some lubes, also, can represent the danger of a condom breaking by degrading the latex these are made of. Most of you reading this are in long-term relationships, so I'm assuming you're not using these, but one never knows. It's good information to have at your disposal.

Silicon-based

This type of lube is beloved by many for its texture, which has a sensual, silken quality. Also, extremely good for those with sensitive skin are that silicon-based products that are hypoallergenic. Lubricants made with silicon are also known for their long duration. That means you'll have "re-load" less frequently than you might with a water-based lube.

All that said, the one thing about this type of lube is that it's not advisable for use with sex toys that are made of silicon, as this can cause the material to deteriorate. But take heart, because silicone-based lubricants are ideal for use when you and your love are going aquatic. In the shower, tub, lake, river or hotel swimming pool, silicone-based lubricants are ideal for water sports.

Hybrids

Just like the cars! Hybrids are a little bit water and little bit silicon, which means they can use them in water, too. While maintaining the naturalism of water-based products, they maintain the quality of longer duration that silicon-based products are known for. As with the 100% silicon type of lube, though, these are not good for use with any toys you might have, if you want to keep them in the best possible shape.

Oil-based

Some people really enjoy the sensation of an oil-based lube. Also good for sensitive skin, the heavier quality of an oil-based product can be uniquely sensual. That said, these lubes are not great for use with condoms. Latex doesn't much like oil. As said above, my long-term relationship readers may or may not care about this detail, but it's important safety information I feel it's responsible to include here.

Another important point about oil-based products is that they make a mess. So, if you're a fan, you may want to lay a couple of towels down on the bed before you get rolling.

If you've never used a sexual lubricant before, experiment with quantities. Start with a little and add more, if the two of you feel you need it. A little dab will do you isn't just for hair gel or pomade. This maxim applies equally to lube. It's not exactly cheap, so start small and work your way up from there.

Personally, I'm a huge fan of hybrid lubes for their versatility. My partner and I are water sport enthusiasts, especially when we visit our favorite vacation rental (in an unnamed land), which features a private dipping pool. There's nothing like cooling off after a hot day at the beach with a hot evening in the dipping pool, a refreshing beverage and a side of long duration lubricant. For our toys, though (which we'll talk about shortly), we always use the time-honored water-based lubricant, as we like our toys and want them to enjoy long, happy lives.

My love and I are also fans of any product that warms upon application, as these can add an entirely new dimension to sex play. These are offered over a wide variety of product lines and price points. I suggest you do your research and find the one that's most appealing. Another "best practice" for happy couples everywhere, is carrying portable lubes. These are sachets that can be carried in your wallet or purse and put to work wherever you may be when the mood strikes you. Well worth the small investment required, these babies come in mighty handy in a pinch.

Lube is a chemical substance subject to deterioration in extreme temperature conditions, so like perfume, make sure to store it in a place which is subject to few fluctuations in temperature. You may find that you've soon accumulated a "lube cellar", so give your personal lubricant the respect it deserves and it'll be ready for playtime when you and your love need it.

Where to buy it

You can buy personal lubricants pretty well anywhere, including on the internet. A trip to your local megastore or drugstore could send you home with what you need, too. A trip to Costco could send you home with enough of it for the entire neighborhood! But where's the fun and adventure in such mundane solutions?

I have a better idea!

You and your love will go on a shopping expedition. Every town on the map, these days, features at least one sex shop within shooting distance. If yours is a particularly pokey little town, with only one horse and no such retail outlets, then perhaps a weekend getaway to the nearest outpost of Western Civilization is in order? Re-discovering the passion you once shared as a couple is all about adventure and this could be one more. Plan your excursion, whether it's in your town, or to a nearby city. Make a shopping list together. Plan your adventure as you would any other excursion.

Once you've decided on the type of lube you'd like to experiment with, write it at the top of the list. I'm about to add to that list, with my personal recommendations of some of the best sex toys and "peripherals". These recommendations are all based on personal preference and incorporate the input of my love, because we've been on more than one such shopping expedition. We love doing this, from time to time, whether in search of something new, to find a specific product, or just to replenish our "lube cellar".

Let's jump into the world of sex toys with both feet. I was once a newbie in the land of the battery-operated sex prop, so if you're shy, I understand. It was, in fact, my adventurous partner who first dragged me into this exciting world and so, I'm returning the favor and inviting you along. Load in those batteries, kids! You're going to need them.

Chapter 12: So you want to be a Superhero?

What do women really want? Well, the answer to that question really isn't all that complicated. Women know when they've pleased a man. They can visually see the pleasure, feel the pleasure and even taste the pleasure they are giving to a man. For men, it's harder to truly identify whether or not the woman they are with has received a great deal of pleasure or any at all, unless of course, she squirts. Women have been known to fake an orgasm just to act like their man has pleased them to that level. But why make a woman fake something when you can actually make her reach that point? Pleasing a woman really isn't that difficult, you just have to give your woman the time and attention that she needs in order to really be able to identify what she likes. DON'T RUSH ANYTHING; MAKE SURE YOU GIVE YOUR WOMAN AS MUCH TIME AS SHE NEEDS!

Many women may be shy or even insecure about what they like. They may have a difficult time telling a man what they want him to do to her. The reality is that while yes, women need to open up and start being honest about this, men also need to encourage the process. Having the initial conversation is crucial. When a woman knows that her man really cares about how she feels and wants her to feel pleasure, she will be more inclined to tell him what will help her feel this way. As a man, you need to tell your woman that you want her to have an orgasm and that you want to pleasure her. This may seem obvious but you must verbalize this wish. Ask her what she likes, do it through text messages or over the phone if it's too difficult in person. Text messages and phone calls have actually helped sexual relationships as they relieve some of the tension when trying to have a face to face conversation about what each individual wants sexually. Actually, text messages can really spice things up and get your girl in the mood. Even a random text message of what you want to do to her can help turn her on. You should not rely to heavily on technology to aid you in your sex life though. At the end of the day face-to-face interaction is the best way to communicate, obviously.

If you really want to make a girl have an orgasm, you have to be ready to try different things in order to help her get there. It can be difficult for some women to have an orgasm, but this is a time when you have to be all about pleasuring her and not yourself. This is difficult for some men. Some men are overwhelmed with the need to have an orgasm and they forget to worry about whether or not their woman received pleasure as well. A real man, or a superhero for that matter will want the woman to have an orgasm over himself. He will make sure that she is pleasured before he allows himself to have an orgasm. While some things are out of the control of the man, such as having a premature orgasm, he will still focus on pleasing his woman first. I've personally had one man ejaculate while he was performing cunnilingus on me. The sound of me moaning during my orgasm was enough to set him over the edge. This just goes to show that sexual pleasure has a lot to do with the mind.

One thing that really encourages most women to have an orgasm is cunnilingus. Women dream, fantasize and think about this often. Cunnilingus for a woman is a time where the woman can literally just lay back and feel pleasure without having to do anything. That being said, this can be a difficult task for a man. The man must try different things with this to really see what his woman likes. Ask for feedback while performing this action, ask her if it feels good, move around, move her legs, pull her to the edge of the bed, try different things until you find the perfect spot. Cunnilingus doesn't have to just be done alone, try using your hands with this as well. When you involve both your fingers and your tongue, your woman is more likely to achieve a full, mind-blowing orgasm. Try one finger first and two if you feel the need, while still maintaining the movement you are doing with your tongue. Really focus on where your fingers are and where your tongue is. While you want to first start by licking all around, you then want to focus on her special spot if you really want her to have an orgasm. Licking that area enough, fast and slow will help her get there. Many women enjoy the sensation of being licked on their anus. Talk about this with your woman and give it a try if you're both think it would be enjoyable.

Once she has an orgasm, you don't need to stop there. In fact, you may even be able to please her twice. Let her cool off for a minute. Right after a woman has an orgasm, she may be a bit sensitive, ticklish even. Give her a few minutes. Try washing your face after this to give her a chance to get cool off and get ready for round two. Washing your face after this will most likely allow for kissing to take place after this is done. This may not be necessary for some women, but others will definitely appreciate it, especially if she's a squirter!

Once you've given her some time, come back and start kissing her. Let her know by telling her that you want to make her have another orgasm. Now, it may be easier for her to have an orgasm by riding you or it may be easier for her to have an orgasm if you're on top. Whatever she wants, give it to her. Before you go in again however, start with more foreplay to get her bodily fluids flowing once more. Start by kissing her softly, kiss her neck, her breasts, even her stomach but don't touch her yet. Let her know that you want her again but give her some time to build the anticipation up again. Foreplay is really important during the time right after she has an orgasm, as it will encourage the likelihood of her having a second orgasm.

Get her in the mood. Gently caress her legs up and down without touching her and let her feel you. This is a soft, sensitive moment, don't rush it. When she feels you, this alone will turn her own. Show her how hard you are. She may even suck you a little but don't let her allow you to orgasm, remember you want her to go again! When a woman goes down on a man this is often a huge turn on for her! Keep in mind, this may be different for all women but many women are incredibly turned on by their man's erect penis in their mouth.

When a man is erect and a woman feels this, it will most likely turn her on and she will start to think about what it will feel like inside of her. If you're lucky, she'll kiss you and lick you just enough to get you even harder than you were before. If she starts going too fast and you feel like you won't last long, pull her off of you a little and bring her up to your mouth so you can kiss her. When you stop her from making you have an orgasm, you'll make her want you even more because she'll know that you're really in it to let her feel more pleasure, not just for her to make you have an orgasm and that be the end of it.

Once you feel like she's ready for you, place her in the position that you know will help her achieve an orgasm. This may vary but find the most likely position and go at it. If you don't know, ask her. Straight out ask her where she wants you and how she wants it. She may hop on all fours and show you what she wants. Once again, you won't know unless you ask, so ask away!

Chapter 13: Develop Sexual Intuition

An INSTINCT is a kind of inner force that drives us to act in a certain way to satisfy it ... therefore, the sexual instinct is an inner force, something like an accumulation of energy, which impels us to release it through a practice sexual. While in the rest of the animal species this works exactly like this, in people it varies a little, because the instinct is mixed with other things that influence it.

Thus, among animals, instinct is present as a guarantee of procreation and, consequently, of the conservation of the species, and does not seem to have any other known purpose. Its activation is biological, mediated mainly by the increase of a series of specific hormones, and when it occurs, with cyclical character, gives rise to the so-called period of estrus, which results in the non-deliberate search for sexual partners and copulation, which occurs repeatedly until the activation ceases (the heat).

Among people, the activation of the sexual instinct also has a biological component, mediated by the presence of specific hormones but, above all, by some other factors, such as an image, a thought, an odor, or a slight touch, a dream ... and this is so, because among people the purpose of sexuality is not only procreation but also that of obtaining pleasure, which is produced through the liberation of the energy of which we spoke earlier.

When a man sees a beautiful woman pass by, the reason is hidden. The sexual instinct in man is more developed than in any other animal, so do not say that we act like animals, these normally act in times of reproduction, while a man at all times, because it is more constant since it has much more energy without losing its intensity. In this way it can reach certain sexual abnormalities since its fixations increase, degenerating in its actualization towards any cultural end. Each person is different instinctively, which can be caused by the way of life or how educated. Speaking of sex education, for most societies, in which we live above all we have sought a certain measure of sexual satisfaction, which is one of the social injustices, where a cultural standard required of all individuals for an equal sexual behavior, on which they are based, is good for a person who holds power with a physical constitution that is puny. It is a laugh since the best constituted can suffer a psychic sacrifice. Although it is very difficult that this type of injustice is mostly fulfilled and any moral precept goes down the drain.

It can not be argued that there are people with a sexual instinct that is too intense, that surpasses many, that extreme perversity is manifested and that if it continues in that role, it must bear the consequences of its cultural divergence, otherwise it can reach an inhibition by the demands social results in an unsatisfied satisfaction, by those substitution phenomena caused by inhibition of their instincts, which can cause a series of mental disorders, a continuous internal impoverishment, which will lead to a harmful form for the person.

In the sexual instinct, its purpose is pleasure manifested from childhood, through its erogenous zones and can dispense with another erotic object in the form of autoerotism, so many people with that energy suffer through the culture that repression of the elements of sexual arousal. The sexual abstinence in both sexes has been forgotten, it can be affirmed and argued that there is no harm whatsoever of any person who makes sex before marriage has any consequence, rather what must be accepted is that there is no means to to be able to dominate this powerful impulse that is the sexual instinct, is very strong and less in that fiery stage as it is the youth. To remove that toy takes them as I said before, to a mental disorder, some erase of neurosis, like those suffered by women, but this has changed. In them, this has stopped being "endure" many calamities of man and the roles are reversed in some points, there is no or very little that nervousness caused by marital infidelity, now the nervous man. This severity towards the woman in this cultural exigency is the sexual instinct begins to disappear her desires and fantasies emerge, they do not remain in the neurosis.

The sex trade is broader, more open; Innocence begins to end, temptations are too many. And the impulses got bigger. Abstinence is only left as a word, before it was preferred to virgin women at marriage because the man in his machismo wanted, according to him, to teach them in the trade of their pleasure or to be the first in his life. Some people presume their abstention, but it is a lie, this is supplemented by other means such as masturbation or analogous practice.

This type of activity seems harmless but in the long term can cause a mental disturbance, although beforehand in our culture masturbation is still subject to attack by that existing morality that leads to a custom to keep on that easy path of not fighting for some sexual object where you can develop your energy. That comfort of a small effort that satisfies your fantasies, can deteriorate in your sexual effort because when you want to translate that fantasy to reality it can be difficult.

Men who have this sexual practice, onanistic or perverse can cause their libido to change and at the time of their sexual potential development can be diminished. Just as women who have retained their virginity until marriage, for that sex education imposed by ceasing to have pleasure and when they overcome that artificial delay to their sexual development and reach the peak of their female existence, one can find that relationships with her partner has cooled down a while ago and there is no other way for them to be that unsatisfied desire, infidelity or a kind of neurosis. If these types of people join, what they can cause is a decrease in their erotic faculties, a lack of potential on the part of man and dissatisfaction in both that would weaken the relationship.

An unsatisfied sexual behavior can cause an effect on the children, from an exaggerated tenderness, concentrating on them that need for love which would cause an anticipated sexual maturity. Due to the disagreement of the couple, the child experiences a series of passions such as hatred, jealousy, love which awakens their sexual activity at an early age, which causes a conflict that manifests itself in nervousness that can last all the time. Lifetime.

There is no person who has become ill due to sexual satisfaction, but because of sexual restrictions under the demands of an imposed sexual morality, stagnant libido becomes dangerous and causes illness.

In the same situation, you can not force a couple to a satisfaction through a limited number of populations, as to use that range of ways of making sex that can lead to unfamiliar pleasures, either by fear of another experience or certain complex taxes when you do not want to change, in this aspect you can disappear several things, from the tenderness of the deprivation of sex they turn to another type of illusion, but that usually leads them to that state of domination and deviation of the sexual instinct, promulgating that series of restrictive precepts for society that living in that "double" moral makes believe that they are fulfilled.

Limiting sexual activity increases more factors that disturb the individual's capacity for enjoyment, desire is reduced, fear of life increases and fear of death increases. That sacrifice that is demanded or rather that is imposed by that sexual morality together with other restrictions is restricting freedom and individual happiness.

Chapter 14: Sexual Massages

Massage and sex go together like red wine and chocolate. If you are stressed out and your muscles are tense, blood flow to your genitalia will be compromised, making sexual arousal nearly impossible. To combat this issue, we highly recommend you incorporate some erotic massage into your romance repertoire. A good sexual experience cannot happen unless you wake up your sexual energy and allow it to both flow and build.

However, having a massage manual open on one side of the bed, and stopping intermittently to read a set of instructions is not going to make for the hottest of massages. Anything that takes you out of the moment and keeps you from "Being Here Now" is a turn off to your erotic energy, and stopping to read an instruction manual is definitely an "off."

Unless you are highly experienced at giving erotic massages, even trying to memorize a series of massage techniques is distracting for the massage giver, as you focus mentally on the list of techniques in your head instead of focusing on the touch, taste and scent of your partner. Your partner will feel consciously or unconsciously that you are in your own head, and not totally "Here."

The answer is an auditory guided massage. An audio track that smoothly takes you from one massage technique to another, without the distraction of reading or remembering. A guided massage, so long as it's slow and smooth, allows you to "Be Here Now," and just enjoy and revel in the sensations.

Several years ago we found a wonderful video by acclaimed sexologist Jaiya (yes, like Cher and Madonna, it is apparently just Jaiya), who had created a guided massage video called "Erogenous Zones and Orgasmic Massage" as part of her "Red Hot Touch" video series.

We had intended to describe how guided erotic massage could be used in your love play, and to point you to this great video. However, sadly the video is apparently no longer available (and no, you can't borrow our copy). We then scoured the internet looking for similar guided massages, and unfortunately, everything we found was terrible.

Guided massages have been for us a wonderful way to build erotic energy, and have been part of some of our best sensual experiences. We didn't want you to miss the opportunity to enjoy this, so we decided if you can't find it, make it!

While the sensual but tasteful video portion of Jaiya's video is instructive, we found that it is not really necessary, and that an audio-guided massage is totally adequate. To that end, we made and used our own guided massage audio, and the script to this is found at the end of this book. For us it was even better than Jaiya at building our erotic energy. After all, we made it to our own sexual tastes! You can create your own audio-guided massage, using the script found near the back of this book in "Appendix: Erotic Guided Massage Script" or by adapting it to your own particular pleasures. Simply read the script, slowly and sexily and with the appropriate pauses, into a recording device like your smartphone and then play it back for both of you via a blue tooth speaker and enjoy an erotic massage experience. The script we have written will result in an approximately 40-45 minute massage, but of course, you can adapt it to be longer or shorter to your pleasure.

Creating your own guided erotic massage will take some effort, but isn't that a great gift to give your lover, letting them know how much you care about their pleasure? You may find, as we did, that just making the guided massage and imagining it as you go is a stimulating experience and a bit of foreplay on its own. We hope you also find that actually doing your own erotic massage leads to some incredible, incendiary sex, just as we did.

One final note on this topic. We know that as we age, our stamina and hand strength can diminish, and for those with arthritis in their hands, this may be especially true. Don't feel like you have to commit to a long full-body session. Even mini five-minute sessions can provide tremendous comfort and pleasure. One area to focus on is the buttocks and upper thighs. We all carry a lot of tension in these areas and helping to ease this will greatly increase blood flow to the genital region, thus allowing for more sexual arousal. One great tip we learned from Jaiya is that the gluteal fold (the crease under your butt cheeks) is actually quite a powerful erogenous zone. Spend some time rubbing and pressing along that area on your partner's body. You may be surprised by the results!

Types of massage to try on your partner

Look into your partner's eyes when you start touching his genitals. Make sure that the connection you made at the beginning of the massage still exists; if it does not, try to restore it by slowing down and asking your partner some questions about what he or she is experiencing. When continuing the genital massage, remember to use your free hand to tease the rest of your partner's body.

Female genital massage
Start by gently rubbing the entire vulva, following with clitoral stimulation, and finishing with internal and clitoral stimulation - do not forget the G-spot! Vaginal penetration can only take place in case of a fairly extreme level of awakening. If your partner is comfortable, feel free to use a vibrator to help you with the massage.

Male genital massage
Begin by applying a lubricant into the palm of your hands and gently applying it to the penis and testicles. Male genital massage is guided by one essential principle: to slow down and stop or change what you

are doing just before ejaculation becomes inevitable. Keep him on the verge of ejaculation as much as possible. Ask your partner to let you know if he is about to ejaculate, which may have the effect of making him enjoy immediately if he is too excited or develops a signal - Change the pace. Play with the brake, caress him, and tickle him.

The massage is nearing completion. By bringing your partner to the extreme limit without allowing him to ejaculate, you prolong the massage and help him to have a more intense orgasm, powerful, if he wishes it.

Sensual or erotic massages
Sensual massage, erotic massage, body-body, and sexual massage are relaxing massages but can go beyond relaxation and well-being. This massage is very different from a traditional massage.

It involves good communication with the other, in a mutual spirit of trust and abandonment. It is sensual in the sense that the gestures are more caresses with a strong erotic tendency. These caresses are worn all over the body, including - but not only - on the genital and intimate parts, for the pleasure and enjoyment of the person who receives them.

This massage is very gradual to appreciate the continuous rise of pleasure better, and intermediate levels are established to slow down and enjoy more of the moment and increase desire.

The pleasure of the person being massaged is the main objective of this massage which can enter the game of caresses not only with the hand, the fingers but also the lips, the tongue, tissues or any other thing contributing to this excitement.

Because some people need to feel the desire of the other to feel theirs better and to express it better, the masseur will let himself be wholly undressed or even suggest to continue with a body-body massage.

Also, some people wishing to go further penetrations will accept the use of their stimulators, their intimate toys or the active participation of the masseur, his fingers, his tongue, his hooded sex, then leading to sex massage.

Body to body massage
This massage is exceptional. It is incredibly erotic and supposes the active participation of the two people who become in turn part of the massage of the other. It is

practiced naked, body to body. The body of each is put to contribution, and it is not only hands that massage but the whole body, from head to toe. It implies a willingness to give as much as to receive.

Although the genitals are thus laid bare, it is not a matter of making banal sexual intercourse. On the contrary, the intensity of this massage is stronger when the couples agree to practice it without sexual penetration despite the natural and visible excitement of the moment. This does not prevent the two people involved in this massage to feel desire, or even to enjoy intensely.

In conclusion, on a table nearby, have sweets: fresh fruit, chocolates, and why not champagne in an ice bucket? Choose soft music that invites you to tenderness. If you like the smell, burn incense.

Chapter 15: Mindful Oral Sex

Every man thinks he's a master when it comes to his mouth—whether this refers to his apparent storytelling skills down at the pub or going down on a woman. But in reality, only the men who know that there's no such thing as "being the best at giving head" can lay legitimate claim to that title—because whereas there are basic rules, each woman will get off on a slightly different technique to the next. And even once you've got it right with the woman you're with, sticking with the same old technique time after time is like giving her a red rose every year for Valentine's Day—nice but lacking imagination. I'll give you ideas that can help make the difference between reaching that climax peak and having to remain in the shadows of the mountain, never quite getting to the top.

Finding Your Way

Knowing your route, how long it'll take and what to look for once you've arrived are essential aspects of a well-executed journey—in this section, we'll address ways to make your oral road to her orgasm a smooth one.

Don't go down too early

Heading down there at high speed is like putting her dessert on the table before you've served appetizers and the main course. She may be looking forward to the dessert more than anything else, but she'll want the savory experience, too—it provides a buildup and makes the end of the meal even sweeter. An orgasm is the release of sexual tension, so the more you build that tension, the greater the eventual release will be.

It's also about intimacy; once your head has disappeared down below and she's left with the sight of your forehead for company, it can be a bit disconcerting, especially if you've only been kissing and touching for a short time. But what constitutes a "short" time? That depends on the woman, but here's an easy way to check if she's ready: if you've been kissing her breasts and nipples and she hasn't been pulling you back up to kiss her lips, start a journey with your hands. Let one hand work its way to her vulva—if she's not ready for clitoral stimulation yet, she'll move away or bring your hand back up. If she lets your hand roam free, gradually work your other hand to take over the work your mouth was doing on her breasts, setting your face free to venture south.

Note: As always, sex rules are there to be broken: 95 percent of the time, waiting until she's fully warmed up before heading down is your best bet, but if you're enjoying the kind of red-hot passion session that causes shirt buttons to fly and stockings to be ripped, then rapidly raising her skirt to feast might be just the thing.

When she's not quite to your taste

This is every woman's nightmare, the thought that she might not smell or taste quite right and so you might not be so enthusiastic when you're down there; worse, you might never go down there again.

To avoid any bad feelings, you need to somehow "taste the waters" before it's too late (worst-case scenario is to go delving with your tongue, then rapidly pull away). If you find her smell or taste unpleasant, there's no point in trying to fake it—if she's in any doubt about your enthusiasm to be down there, she'll be wondering what's wrong, which means she won't orgasm. The result? You'll be stuck down there even longer! So use your fingers down there first, then give them a sniff or a lick when you're kissing her neck so she can't see what you're up to. If it doesn't smell fresh enough for your taste, you have two choices: avoid going down there during this bedroom session or suggest a shower. And if you go for the shower option, make sure you make it about getting sexy rather than getting clean: "Shall we do it in the shower?" rather than "Let's go and wash before we get down to it."

What is a normal smell?

It's important here to differentiate between a woman's natural smell and bad vaginal odor. The former is musky, like a more subtle, warmer, and sweeter version of fresh underarm sweat; the latter is like bad breath, rancid and unnatural smelling. The musky odor has a purpose: scientists believe that one of the reasons we still have hair between our legs and under our arms is to capture and enhance our genetic odor—it's a way of giving each other genetic information without having to chat about our ancestry or medical history. Pubic hair also helps protect the genitals from infection by creating a hairy barrier to liquids that could otherwise be absorbed. But don't be duped into believing that removing the hair will remove any odors; far from it, it might make them worse. Removing her pubes could disrupt the natural pH balance of the vagina and can expose her genitals to bacteria that might otherwise be held at bay.

Getting past her hair and lips

Some women are confident enough to spread their legs wide and let you in; others aren't. If you can't get full access or her lips are getting in your way, put your hands to good use.

Getting past her hair and lips

Some women are confident enough to spread their legs wide and let you in; others aren't. If you can't get full access or her lips are getting in your way, put your hands to good use.

Gently slide your hand down her stomach and onto her thigh, easing it away from the other one—this will open up her vaginal lips a little. Now, keep using your hands: place your thumb toward the lower end of her vaginal lips (nearer her anus) where her lips usually sit further apart, and slide your thumb upwards to her belly button, use your other hand to help hold the other lip to one side. This clears the path to her clitoris just like a plow through a field of earth—now follow your thumb with your tongue to find that precious seed at the top of the trough.

Still can't find her clitoris?

If you're licking her all over her lips in an effort to find her pleasure point, don't panic. At this stage she doesn't realize you don't know where it is, she just thinks you're one of the rare (and wonderful) men who spend time exploring and learning about her vulva before heading straight for the clitoris. Some women have huge visible clitorises—the size of a broad bean—others have such tiny ones, you wouldn't bother eating it if it were a pea. But all women have thousands of nerve endings in their vaginal lips as well as that little clitoral button—so explore away, you're getting her well-oiled for the drive of a lifetime.

If you're desperate to get into that driving seat but still can't locate the clitoral gearshift, there is a foolproof way to find it. All women have two outer lips and two inner—they're large and small, fat and thin, never the same and almost never look like the genitals of porn stars who have usually had cosmetic surgery. Start licking at the bottom of her lips, where her vagina is (her vagina isn't the entire genital area, as is often thought, but the "hole" where your penis goes during penetrative sex), and get your tongue between her inner lips. As you slide your tongue from the bottom toward the top—in the direction of her pubic mound or her belly button—you'll reach a point where the lips meet. This is like the corner of your mouth. It's in this area, the "upper corner" of her genital mouth, where you'll find the clitoris.

And if you still can't pinpoint that sexually explosive pea, concentrate your entire tongue on this upper corner—let your tongue flatten against your chin as you grind your face on the entire area. This technique works well for a lot of women because even if the clitoris can't be seen or felt, it's still receiving plenty of stimulation from the pressure your face provides.

When the going gets tough...
Women are, by and large, caring creatures, and so if you've been down there for what feels like forever to you, it's likely she realizes it's taking a while and that'll make her less able to relax...which means she's less likely to come.

Technique

The longest, strongest tongue won't cut the mustard with any woman unless you know how to use it. Rhythm, pressure, speed, variation, and pattern, and all-important saliva, are what you need to be thinking about. And that's what I'll help you do right now.

Easy on the pressure

The clitoris is not a magic button that must be found at all costs and pressed repeatedly until you get her orgasmic bells ringing—the clitoris head is even more sensitive than your penis and some women simply can't handle having it touched directly. It is, however, the key to her orgasm—a woman cannot orgasm without stimulation to her clitoris (scientists believe that even a "vaginal orgasm" occurs through stimulation of the clitoris, but via the "arms" that extend back into her body rather than the head that's visible), but the stimulation needn't be direct. While masturbating, women may use the palm of their hand, a flat vibrator, or even a pillow—this allows for stimulation of the entire area, lips included, without putting too much pressure directly on the clitoris. So how can you simulate that in the bedroom? Easy—use your mouth and chin, and bring your tongue out only for the occasional flat pressure-lick. By using your lips, you can't apply the same zoned pressure on her clitoris as you could with your tongue (try it on your hand and you'll see), but you'll still be providing ample stimulation to the entire region—plenty to bring her to orgasm. Be thankful; pressing your lips into her vulva rather than having to use your tongue on her clitoris will save you a lot of tongue ache. Good news for her, too—that means you'll be able to engage in some post-sex talking.

Practice makes perfect

Keeping up a constant pressure and rhythm is no mean feat—but the tongue, just like any part of the body, can be worked on to become fitter and stronger. Midori, a world-renowned sex teacher, shows her pupils how to perfect oral technique by using fruit as well as a mint candy (you'll have to ask her about that one). She suggests using a plum to strengthen your tongue muscles—you simply keep licking and applying pressure until the skin breaks. Then once you've broken through, you've got to find your way to the plum's stone and get it out! Do that regularly and your muscles will grow to be big and strong.

And, just as you would after eating a plum, lick your lips after going down on a woman, don't wipe. That's the gentlemanly—and very sexy—thing to do.

Forget about licking the alphabet

This old trick has been written about in several sex books and magazines, but I'm yet to meet a woman who says it'll bring her to orgasm. There is a small possibility that she'll climax by having the alphabet licked onto her clitoris, but chances are it will be interesting, exciting even, for no more than a half a minute or so—as a teaser—quite quickly it will feel rather frustrating, like being in bed with a man who has to change sex position after every thrust. Keep the alphabet trick for times you'd like to play with her or get her aroused, but don't rely on it to bring her to orgasm, as you're unlikely to succeed.

Use your hands, too

Ever enjoyed a woman's hands squeezing your behind while giving you oral? Ever reached climax as she's played with your nipples while sucking you? Ever been sent over the edge as she's handled your balls while going down? Well, what a coincidence—women also like to be touched when a man goes down on them. Trouble is, most men (and women when the roles are reversed) are so focused on the task in hand—their tongue and lips and her lips and clitoris—that they forget she even has a body with plenty of other erogenous zones that will bring her to a more explosive orgasm sooner.

Try any of these hands-on approaches:

Start at the bottom. Grab her behind to give yourself better access and extra stimulation power—you can push up as you lick down, maximizing the effects of your tongue or lips.

Find her breasts. If you have long enough arms to play with her love pillows at the same time as giving her oral, you'll be rewarded with plenty of brownie points.

Press on her mons pubis.

That's the bony pubic area above her vagina. Don't do it hard, but if you pull the flesh back here you expose her clitoris and many women really enjoy the sensation.

Don't forget her hands. Grabbing her hands is a nice intimate thing to do when you're giving her oral, plus it also gives you extra control—you can pull her body down onto your face if you have both of her hands in yours.

Techniques to bring her to orgasm quicker

Use one of the following moves when you go down on her, but don't forget to experiment: try variations of each and make up new techniques!

The no-move move

Simply hold your tongue firm and let her do the moving and shaking. As sex therapist Dr. Ian Kerner puts it, "A flat, still tongue is one of the most underestimated oral-sex techniques." And he's so right. If women most enjoyed flicking, darting tongues, they'd invest in a lizard—have you ever even seen a sex toy designed to look like one? No. That's because they prefer a firm, even pressure. Hold your tongue and you'll hold the key to her orgasm.

Chapter 16: Alternative Sexual Experiences

For most people, threesomes, bondage, and anal sex only happen in movies. They don't have to be sequestered into the fantasy realm. With some planning, you can make your anal sex, bondage, or threesome a very sexual reality. Here is how.

Threesomes

If you have a partner that you are comfortable with, you need to pick your third partner carefully. It is a lot more complicated than staying away from best friends or ex-lovers. Relationship and sex experts say that finding one person in your friend group that you aren't that close to but is open to having a threesome. If you choose a stranger, you don't have to worry about long-term attachments, but you do risk not being attracted to the person you are getting ready to have sex with. There are also some safety hazards to take into consideration like sexually transmitted diseases.

If you are single, try dating sites that cater to people that are looking for multiple partners like POF. This also goes for Craigslist. Craigslist has a tendency to attract some weird people so you might want to FaceTime with them or meet them in person in a group setting first. There are some other sites like 3nder and FetLife that are interesting. You could always go to your local sex toy store and talk with people there. You could ask the people who work there or the owners what happens in the community and you might even find some fliers for other clubs or parties.

It doesn't matter if it is two women and a man or two men a one woman, it is totally up to you either as an individual or couple. Male-female-female is most common since guys are as open-minded about being with another man. With that said, women shouldn't cave just because her partner is forcing his preference on her.

If you haven't discussed this with your partner, you might need to suggest watching a movie about threesomes before outright asking your partner about having one. Once you see their reaction to the movie, you can ask them if they have had one or would be interested in having one.

If it goes well, you might casually ask them if they have anyone in mind to be their third. If you both agree to the person, then you need to approach them in a way, so you don't scare them off. Ask them casually like, "Hey, we think you are cool and fun. We would like to have a threesome, and we think we would have a lot of fun with you. Would you be interested?" If you already know the person, let them know that this will not change the friendship in any way. If it is someone you don't know, take time to get to know them first. Go out to dinner or drinks to see if you have a connection with them and feel like you can trust them.

Don't worry so much about asking. Most people on the receiving end will feel flattered.

You need to set some ground rules well in advance. You could think about taking sleepovers, oral sex, kissing, or possibly penetration off the table. Don't worry about taking activities off the table will make the experience worse, it could actually be more exciting without actually penetrating.

If you are in a relationship, you and your significant other could set up safe words or phrases you could use if things start to get too intense. Let the third person know they can speak up if they ever feel uncomfortable.

There are some things you need to have on hand. You are going to need plenty of condoms. If the man is penetrating each woman, he will need to take the condom off every time he changes partners. If he doesn't, he is exposing them to viruses, infections, and bacteria. Sex toys, lube, and toy cleaning wipes need to be on hand for wetness or added sensations. Toys need to be wiped down between partners, so you don't spread germs.

It is all easier said than done. Don't over-think things. Begin with a glass of wine and some appetizers. Start talking, and this will usually lead to flirting. Somebody will make a move in no time.

Massage is a good way to get intimate. There are massage candles that turn into an oil when blown out. This can be used to give a body rub that will set the mood.

The actual three-way needs to be organic. Maneuver, touch, and move any way you like. If you are a dominate person, take the lead. If not, let yourself be led and do what feels natural.

For some positions, the man could lay down on his back and receive oral sex from one partner while the other woman sits on his face and gets oral sex from him. A different position is one woman lies on her back while the other one lies on top of her. The guy penetrates the top woman doggy style, and the women can play with each other. Another option is to arrange everybody in a circle, and everyone performs oral sex on each other.

There are plenty of places to put mouths, genitals, and hands. If there is a free tongue or hand, find a place to put it.

Threesomes will take longer than normal sex, so you might need to change things up a lot. Guide your partners into ways you would like to do. Pay attention to any changes in the other's body language, sexual cues, and breathing patterns. Use movements to guide them, no words.

If it seems like someone is being left out, reach out and begin to play with them. This will help them to jump back in action.

You will need to figure out what you are going to do after the action beforehand. Let the others know. You might want just to say goodbye then, cuddle up for a while, or just hand out. Just remember to talk about what is expected of everyone, so no one is surprised later on. If a sleepover is planned, the third party needs to know in advance so they can pack an overnight bag.

Bondage

If bondage is new to you and your partner, bring up the subject gently, so they won't freak out. During sex, begin by pinning your partner's hands down and telling them that they are now at your mercy. Let this be a starting point to the conversation about pushing the subject of bondage more.

Blindfolds are a great place to start since they don't feel as strange as handcuffs might. Not being able to see will help some get rid of their inhibitions. Take turns blindfolding the other and then treat them to sensations like, kissing, tickling, lightly scratching, and licking your partner in various places, so they don't have a clue as to what is going to happen next. This will mirror the sensations that happen when tying up your partner.

Before you bring out the handcuffs and ropes, you must choose a safe word if things start getting too intense for the submissive. Try the word yellow if you want the dominant one to ease up but not stop. The word red shows your partner that you want to stop completely. The safe word should never be stop or no since saying these things gives the dominant the right to override your protests. Getting your demands overridden is part of the fun of being out of control.

You should only try bondage with someone you feel 100 percent safe with. Now, set a timer for 30 minutes for your first session because it will be extremely intense. Don't use gags or blindfolds for the first few times. Just try tying up the submissive partner, so you learn to read each other. Do not ever leave a person that is tied up alone.

If you think you are ready to push the envelope, start by using a soft rope or silk scarves to tie up your submissive partner up with in different ways. Allow the dominant to configure the rope into a figure eight that goes between the breasts and behind your back. This will push up your breasts and accentuate them. A different scenario has them stand with their arms at their sides and wrap the rope around the torso, so their arms are tied down. Just be creative, let the rope twist over their body any way that feels right. Touch them sexually with your fingers as you pull the rope across and through their body parts. When you finally have them tied up challenge them to escape. Stay away from the neck area. If you decide to tie their ankles together, be sure they can't fall. Never, ever use bungee cords, these will snap and hurt your partner. Don't tie them up too tight. You should be able to slip a finger between the rope and their body. They shouldn't feel any numbness or pain.

The handcuffs you decide to will help to set the tone. Metal or leather will make you feel like a badass where a fuzzy pair will have you feeling playful. Begin by binding your partner's hands together either in front or behind their backs. Move on to a position where they are secured to the bed with their arms up and out to the sides. Never use cheap costume handcuffs. These can tighten and hurt your partner. Don't use stocking as these can cut into the skin.

The dominant partner needs to move into things by starting out sensual and sweet. Think about kissing softly and slowly. It is extremely hot being tied up but yet being treated very tenderly. As the game progresses, the dominant one can bring out their inner tiger.

For another naughty twist, wrap up certain body parts in plastic wrap, like around your hips and breasts. This plastic drives him wild since he will be able to see but not touch you. When you have him good and worked up, allow him to have his way. Have some blunt-tipped scissors near so they can cut you lose.

Another hot idea is to tie your partner up with toilet paper. Be sure to twist it to make it stronger. Tell them they can't break free and then tantalize them until they can't stand it. When they rip loose, then you can punish them.

If you want to take it up a notch, try using a spreader bar. It will hold your partner's legs apart so you can have your way with them.

Role-playing can help transition into bondage. A few fun games are: pirate/princess, prison guard/prisoner, cop/robber, burglar/defenseless housewife.

The biggest part of what makes bondage so pleasurable is the aspect of not allowing your partner to have pleasure. If they are tied up, begin by slowly stripping in front of them. Let them watch as you touch yourself. When they are begging you to touch them, begin by slowly stroking their most intimate parts and then penetrate them slowly. Tell them that they can't have an orgasm until you tell them to.

If both partners agree to be both dominant and submissive, switch between these roles, and you will be amazed at what will get you going.

Anal

Of all the numerous sex acts, Anal remains the most misunderstood. Anal sex is not the first thing when you think about mutually pleasurable things you want to do with your partner. The urban legend states that "Guys want it since they think it is tighter than a vagina. They have seen it in porn, and women use it as a bargaining chip for special occasions."

Quite frankly, that is pure crap. A lot of women do it just because they like it.

The main thing other women want to know is will it hurt?

All women will agree that yes, it does hurt the first few times. The main thing to remember is to relax. Don't think about it. Prepare for it. It won't be as bad if you begin with lube and fingers. Widening the hole before penetration can help it not hurt as bad.

Why do you want to do it?

Mostly because it is considered to be taboo and naughty. Some do it to impress the guy they are with after a night of partying. Having anal sex when you are extremely turned on is more pleasurable. Some women can have an orgasm during anal sex. The ones who do orgasm during anal, say it is more intense than a normal orgasm.

Who wants it more, the woman or man?

Most women say that their men were the ones who initiated anal sex. Most women concede due to the fact they don't want to hurt their men's feelings. They don't want their man to think they aren't into them. Some have been lucky, and it was mutually wanted. Most men are infatuated with anal sex and butts.

How does it feel the first time?

It is very weird. It is very tight and unpleasant. It is a bad cramp. Just like you are stretching a muscle that has never been used before. If you can make yourself relax and be prepared, it will be better.

What will it feel like after you have done it for a while?

It makes you feel like you are completely full. Very intense. You learn to adjust just like you did with normal sex. With time, you know what you are going to fill and learn to enjoy it. It won't hurt as bad since you aren't as nervous. The initial penetration will always feel weird, but once you get going, it is enjoyable.

Will it ever feel good?

If the person you are with lets you control the force and speed; it can be quite pleasurable. It also depends on the size of the man's penis. If you can combine it with clitoral and vaginal stimulation, it can feel great.

Is waxing a necessity?

No, most decent guys don't care what a female looks like back there. If you feel more comfortable, then, by all means, go for it.

How soon into a relationship should it happen?

If the guy has a fetish for this sort of thing, it is really hard to hide, and he will bring it up right away. Most will wait six months or more until you have thoroughly enjoyed each other in all other intimate ways.

To lube or not to lube?

If you don't want it to hurt and feel horrible, lots of lube is needed. They type is up to you. Use whatever you have on hand or your favorite. If you find yourself out of lube but have coconut oil on hand, that works just as well.

Will you bleed?

You shouldn't bleed as long as the guy takes precautions and uses lube. If he forces himself into you, it is possible.

Do you need to protect the bed with towels?

Anal sex isn't messier than normal sex. If you are a squirter, or just get extremely wet during sex, then use a towel.

What is the cleanup like?

There isn't any cleanup. Just the normal lube and wetness. The condom is the only thing that needs to be taken off.

Are there certain positions or angles to try?

Most say the doggy style is the easiest and most convenient. Some women find it pleasurable with the girl on top so she can control the pace.

Are condoms still required?

Absolutely, condoms are still and will always be a requirement.

Can you have an orgasm from anal sex alone?

Usually not. If you can stimulate the clitoris along with anal sex, you will probably have an orgasm. Don't worry about it if you can't. It is all about what you feel with your partner and how they make you feel. Just enjoy yourself and have fun.

Chapter 17: Would You Ever?

Sex is an endless kaleidoscope of possibilities. Just when you thought it was all getting a little tired, along comes another wrinkle in your sexual world, to shake things up again.

A wrinkle, or a kink?

Ah, there's that word. Kink is not all whips and chains. Kink can involve fetishization of certain types of clothing, or body parts, or even household objects. (Stop looking at the blender like that). Kink can be role-play, or public sexual behavior. It can be lots and lots of different things. For as many people as there are in this world, there are different types of kink and you know what? With willing partners, it's okay.

Sometimes people are awfully shy about admitting to a kink or fetish. That's because we live in a judgmental world. Something I've learned in my life, though, is that those who judge you are the people who are most likely to have a closet full of secrets; things they kept hidden, out of shame. But their shame is not your problem. Only your shame is your problem and the fact is that kinkiness is the human condition. There's nothing to be ashamed of.

Role play

You're a superstar. You know you are. You and your partner are the same people every day, doing more or less the same things. Sometimes, when the moment's right, it's kind of fun to put aside our day-to-day personas and be someone else for a little bit. At least, I think it is. My partner does too.

We were on vacation at an all-inclusive beach resort when we found out just how much fun role-play can be. We spent that vacation mostly recharging our batteries, poolside. Cradling cool drinks in our languidly lazy (and sun-browned) mitts, we were as indolent as the day was long, refusing to budge, except to dunk ourselves in the pool momentarily, or flag the waiter down.

And it was that waiter that broke the camel's back. My partner, much to my chagrin, couldn't keep her eyes off him. I admit that he was a pleasant-looking guy (OK, he was built like a brick outhouse and had dimples you could stick your finger in up to the first knuckle). Finally, after observing her eyes peeping out over the top of her sunglasses to bore holes into the guy's ass as he walked away one too many occasions, I got a little testy.

"I can see you, you know." I snorted, sarcastically. "You're not invisible!"

Naturally, my partner pretended not to know what I was talking about, directing her attention back to her pulp fiction, poolside reading. As for me, I sat there turning the meaning of my partner's ogling ways over in my mind. After doing so for the better part of the afternoon, I began to formulate a plan.

When it was time to return to our room to shower and get ready for dinner, I pretended to have an errand to run. I wandered around the grounds of the resort for about twenty minutes and when I felt enough time had elapsed, returned to the room. Knocking on the door, I called out, "Room service!"

When my partner arrived at the door, she found me there, frosty cocktail, replete with paper umbrella, on a tray I'd managed to convince one of the guys at the swim-up bar to lend me for the occasion. She'd just gotten out of the shower and had come to the door wearing a towel.

"Oh, pardon me ma'am! I'm so sorry to disturb you." My eyes roved up and down the length of her towel-clad body, as I said this, lingering on her breasts.

My partner's eyebrows shot up, as she cottoned on.

"That's no problem. Do come in". She pulled the door open, still hanging on to the towel. Closing the door behind me, she gestured to the table in the sitting area. "You can put that over there". And so I did. But when I turned around, my partner had dropped the towel to the floor at her feet and it was on.

Without so much as saying a word, I had become my partner's dirty little fantasy, come to life in our hotel room. It was as easy as paying attention to what was going on right in front of me and transforming it into an experience we could share and enjoy together. This is where putting aside uselessly hurt feelings comes into play. Why should you be hurt or even mildly annoyed that your partner sees other people as attractive? This is just a human thing and an indication that your partner is, in fact, still living!

Don't get angry. Get creative. Take that attraction and make it a game you can both get off playing. That's how the smart folks do things.

Bondage

A little light bondage can be very erotic. It just depends where you're both at, as to whether this option is going to work for you. I'm not talking about heavy-duty dungeon play. Then again, that might be your thing (which is another book, entirely). I'm talking about light restraints around the wrists and possibly, the ankles. This can work for either partner. Have a little chat. Find out if this is something your partner may like. I've found that springing things on my partner can work either for or against me, so once again, knowing your partner well is your best sexual tutor. You know who your partner is better than anyone. Let that knowledge be your guide.

Your visit to the sex shop can encompass this aspect of sex play, too. There are even kits available, which include everything from feather ticklers, to satin wrist restraints and blindfolds, to kinky little whips made of soft, non-threatening material. Perhaps making a gift to your partner of one such kit can break the ice. If such a presentation concludes with something else getting broken, there's your answer.

Spanking

Spanking is becoming an increasingly popular activity for fun-loving couples. As with everything else in this book, its two-way street and one which both of you can enjoy giving and receiving. You may want to incorporate it into your role play, with one of you playing the principal to the naughty school girl/boy. Lights! Cameras! Action! You may even need costumes.

Spanking, though, needn't even incorporate any elaborate scenarios, or equipment. The flat of someone's hand and a naked bottom are quite enough. When incorporated into your sex play, a little slap on the bum can be powerfully erotic and you may find that you both become rather fond of the activity. The trick, of course, is knowing when you've gone a little too far. It's important, when engaging in any activity involving restraints or BDSM (bondage, domination, sadism, masochism), that you're both invested with the ability to stop the action if it's going beyond what you're willing to indulge. That means employing a safe word.

A safe word is what you say when you don't like the direction the action is taking. It has to be a word that neither of you would normally say in the course of your love play. For example, "Pythagoras" is a rather good one. Also appropriate might be a word like "cumberbund" (it's not as though either of you is going to be wearing one – generally speaking). Having an agreed-upon safe word in place can also be fun at parties, when you're both ready to leave for the evening, or if you find someone to be a terrific bore, but don't dare say as much to his or her face. You can always explain it away as a type of Tourette's, if it comes off as too "weird".

Conclusion

What a wonder sex can be for a loving couple. When both partners are actively engaged in keeping the flame alive, sex can be the glue that binds them together. When we let that flame die, for whatever reason, our lives together lose something. We become roommates who used to find each other attractive, once upon a time and perhaps forget how that happened.

It can happen to anyone. It doesn't mean there's something wrong with you, or your partner. Letting the fire go out happens to most people, over the course of their relationships, but I'm here to tell you that the condition is not permanent. With some genuine commitment and sustained remedial action, you can light it up again and it won't even take that much effort. It just takes commitment, dedication and the love that's already there, between you and your partner.

That never went anywhere. That love is still there. It's like gasoline, waiting for a match to be dropped on it. Re-learning how to physically express your love is something the two of you can not only talk about, but do. You can do it together. If only one of you is coming along for the ride, then maybe the writing is on the wall. I'm the type of guy, though, who genuinely believes that if the love is real, then the sex is not dead forever. It's just taking a nap and needs a wakeup call.

With your unique, combined creativity as a couple, every day is going to be an adventure. Your willingness to explore and to rediscover the people you fell in love with, will have you falling in love all over again. There was a time when you couldn't keep your hands off each other and that time can be now, if you're willing to do what it takes to make it happen.

My partner and I, like almost every living couple, has been there. We've let the flame go out. But because we know each other so well and because we love each other so deeply, we've been able to not only revive our sexual relationship, we've been able to make it better than it was, even in our earliest days together. As we've grown together we've become stronger and more fully rounded human beings. Experience has taught us many things, as it teaches us all. That's the part about getting older that's beautiful. Life teaches you as you move through it and all that learning can enrich your lives together, emotionally, sexually and spiritually.

Your relationship was born in passion. There's no reason to believe it's not still there. In fact, believing that serves as the cornerstone re-discovering that passion, together. If your love is real, it was built to last and something built to last is worth keeping in the best shape you possibly can.

While life can throw us curveballs, wear us out and squash us down, our response to those challenges is what really makes the whole affair worth living. Being who you are together and who you've always been as a couple, is a shared adventure and sexuality is an important part of that. Whether you're young, old, physically unencumbered, or disabled, your sexuality is an integral part of your humanity. Living that out in all the fullness and joy sex brings to our lives is your birthright and your gift to one another.

I hope you've enjoyed this open, high-spirited discussion about re-discovering sexual passion as a committed couple. More than that, though, I hope you take what I've written here to heart and that you and your partner can put it to the right kind of use – re-igniting the passion in your relationship. By doing that, you can be a light to other couples out there who may be floundering. The quality of your life has changed because of your dedication to each other, you'll stand as an example to others that love is not disposable. It may change, over time. But it's something worth defending and something worth spending the time to reinforce, by giving ourselves fully to each other. We were born for each other. Let's remember that, and live out our love with our bodies, minds and spirits. Let's be the promise we made to one another in the very beginning.

May you re-discover your passion for each other and live as lovers, always.

www.ingramcontent.com/pod-product-compliance
Lightning Source LLC
Chambersburg PA
CBHW070905080526
44589CB00013B/1186